S0-DOQ-392

HEALING
the PAIN

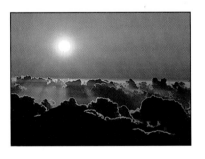

Consultants: Peter J. Vicente, Ph.D.
and Richard V. Gregg, M.D.

Writer: Dianne Molvig

Publications International, Ltd.

Dianne Molvig is a freelance health and medical writer, researcher, and editor whose work has appeared in *Natural Health, Wellness, Parents,* and numerous other publications. She is a contributing author to *Alternative Medicine* and *Your Child's Health: A Medical Record Book.*

CONSULTANTS

Peter J. Vicente, Ph.D., is past president of the American Pain Society and the Midwest Pain Society and is a trustee on the board of CARF, the national standard-setting body for pain and rehabilitation programs. President of Health & Rehabilitation Services, Inc., Dr. Vicente has spent more than twenty years designing, developing, and directing pain-rehabilitation and disability-management programs for public and private hospitals, state government, and other settings. He holds a doctorate in psychology from Ohio State University and is a Diplomate of the American Board of Professional Neuropsychology.

Richard V. Gregg, M.D., completed medical school and internship at the University of Louisville, Kentucky, followed by a residency in anesthesia and a fellowship in pain management at the University of Cincinnati, Ohio, where he served for nine years as director of the pain fellowship program and maintained a practice in pain management. A frequent lecturer on pain, pain control, and pain treatments, Dr. Gregg has contributed to more than two dozen publications on the subject. A former director of the University Pain Control Center at the University of Cincinnati, he is director of the Greater Cincinnati Pain Consortium.

Cover Photo: Frank Cezus/FPG International

Copyright © 1997 Publications International, Ltd. All rights reserved. This book may not be reproduced or quoted in whole or in part by any means whatsoever without written permission from:

Louis Weber, C.E.O.
Publications International, Ltd.
7373 North Cicero Avenue
Lincolnwood, Illinois 60646

Permission is never granted for commercial purposes.

Manufactured in China

8 7 6 5 4 3 2 1

ISBN: 0-7853-2432-1

Note: Neither Publications International, Ltd., nor the authors, consultants, editors, or publisher take responsibility for any possible consequences from any treatment, procedure, exercise, dietary modification, action, or application of medication or preparation by any person reading or following the information in this book. The publication of this book does not constitute the practice of medicine, and this book does not attempt to replace your physician or your pharmacist. Before undertaking any course of treatment, the authors, consultants, editors, and publisher advise the reader to check with a physician or other health care provider.

CONTENTS

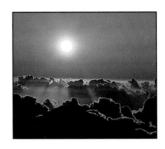

Chapter 17:
Conditions 153

Index 243

INTRODUCTION
Healing the Pain

Pain: We simply don't tolerate it anymore. Although pain used to be an expected and accepted part of life, today it is something we demand to control. Even if we can't eliminate the cause, we believe that modern medicine should be able to vanquish our pain.

Where does that belief come from? The ever-growing pain relief section of your local pharmacy might be partially responsible. Over-the-counter pain relief medications used to take up only a shelf or two. But today an entire section is required to stock all the types and brands of pain relief medications that have been developed. And you can't open a magazine or turn on the television without seeing advertisements touting the remarkable pain relieving capabilities of these nonprescription medications. The number of prescription pain relief medications is also growing, further fueling our assurance that pain control comes in a bottle.

But recent advances in pain management are not limited to medications. In fact, the most important advance is in the way much of the medical community now thinks about pain. Patients are not expected to stoically bear pain, and it no longer is considered an unavoidable companion to illness, injury, and surgery. Many doctors now take pain seriously, understanding that pain itself jeopardizes patients' health in many ways. As a result of this relatively new view of pain, more research is being done to understand its origin and how to treat it. And the medical community has become more open to alternative techniques such as acupuncture and biofeedback, which used to exist only outside mainstream American medical practice.

Whether it's temporary or chronic, mild or severe, when you're in pain you want to know how to stop it. *Healing the Pain* gives you sixteen options for pain management. These techniques range from such conventional treatments as nerve blocks, prescription and nonprescription medication, and the use of cold and heat to such alternative treatments as biofeedback, chiropractic, and hypnosis. In layman's terms we explain the history of each technique, what it is used for, its pros and cons, and research that supports its use. Each chapter ends with advice about how to find a qualified practitioner. The second half of the book is devoted to a discussion of various illnesses that cause pain, such as arthritis and cancer, and the methods that can bring relief.

The purpose of *Healing the Pain* is to acquaint you with the variety of strategies available for managing and/or eliminating your pain. You may find one technique that works, or you may require a combination of several different therapies to achieve adequate relief. The message of *Healing the Pain* is simple: You can control your pain; it doesn't have to control you.

CHAPTER 1
Acupuncture

One legend among many about the origin of acupuncture connects this ancient healing technique to chance discoveries made in the aftermath of battle. According to the legend, Chinese warriors injured by spears later noticed that other, chronic ailments and health problems had mysteriously disappeared. Soon attempts were made to replicate this effect by piercing the body with sharp stones and later with needles made of bone.

THE ASIAN EXPLANATION

Dating back at least 2,500 years and possibly many centuries earlier, acupuncture is one of the oldest medical treatments still used today. It is but one aspect of Chinese medicine, which emphasizes treatment of the whole person, not just a single organ or complaint.

Chinese medicine believes illness to be the result of an imbalance in the body's qi (pronounced "chee"), or life-force energy. This life force has two polarities: yin and yang. Each individual's health depends on maintaining an equilibrium between these two opposing forces.

Qi travels through 14 meridians, or channels, that course through the body. Along these meridians are hundreds of

Healing the Pain

acupuncture points that are considered to be like control switches for the body's qi. Using acupuncture needles, the practitioner manipulates and stimulates these "switches," restoring the energy balance needed for optimum health.

PAIN RELIEF AND MORE

Acupuncture practitioners report that acupuncture can help relieve pain caused by many conditions, including:

- headaches
- temporomandibular joint disorder (TMD)
- muscle strain
- arthritis
- low back pain
- trigeminal neuralgia (severe facial pain)
- tennis elbow
- sports injuries
- fibromyalgia (a migratory muscle-pain syndrome)
- postoperative pain

But acupuncturists use their technique for much more than pain relief. For instance, AIDS symptoms, anxiety, asthma, chronic fatigue syndrome, depression, drug addictions, environmentally induced illnesses, and gastrointestinal problems have all been treated by acupuncturists. In addition, gynecological disorders, infertility, insomnia, menopause symptoms, nausea, nerve degeneration, paralysis from stroke, premen-

Healing the Pain

Coming to America

Although Chinese immigrants brought acupuncture to the United States in the mid-19th century, it wasn't until the early 1970s that it gained widespread attention. Back then, *New York Times* columnist James Reston was covering President Nixon's visit to China. While there, Reston had to undergo an emergency appendectomy, after which Chinese doctors treated his postoperative pain with acupuncture. Reston's accounts of his experience piqued curiosity among many Americans, including several physicians who traveled to China to see for themselves what acupuncture could do.

strual syndrome (PMS), skin conditions, speech disorders, and vision problems also have reportedly responded to this therapy.

WESTERN REACTIONS

For Westerners, the image of piercing the body often triggers an initial aversion, even though modern acupuncturists use thin, stainless-steel needles instead of the primitive instruments used centuries ago. Still, cringing at the thought of acupuncture, the first question Westerners usually ask is, "Does it hurt?" It's certainly a valid question.

Actually, the acupuncturist does not usually insert the needles very deeply—perhaps only a quarter of an inch—and the patient feels little or no discomfort. There may be a slight

Healing the Pain

prickly sensation, or the patient may feel nothing at all; it depends on the individual. In fact, the same person may even feel different sensations on different days or in different parts of the body. When the acupuncturist manipulates the needle by twirling it, the patient may feel a tingling or dull ache. The Chinese refer to this sensation as the *ashi*, or "ah, yes" point, which indicates that the needle is stimulating the movement of *qi*.

Does Acupuncture Work?

After finding out whether it hurts, most people want to know whether acupuncture really works. Westerners accustomed to high-tech medical treatments wonder how simply introducing needles into the body could possibly relieve pain. Explanations about balancing the body's life-force energy have not really satisfied demands by the Western scientific community for proof that acupuncture

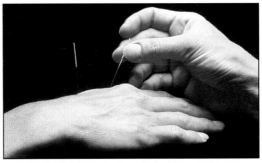

Whether it stimulates the flow of qi or triggers the release of endorphins, the body's natural painkillers, acupuncture does help relieve some painful conditions.

works and, if it does, how. Acupuncture studies proclaiming successful treatment for many health conditions abound in Chinese medical journals. But the research methods employed in these studies rarely, if ever, pass rigorous Western scrutiny.

Healing the Pain

RESEARCH QUANDARIES

Some inherent difficulties exist in efforts to scientifically prove acupuncture's worth:

- Acupuncture practitioners usually haven't been trained in the research methods used in the West.
- Western scientists know little or nothing about Chinese medicine and acupuncture. This may hinder their efforts to set up effective studies.
- The double-blind study is the standard method for studying medical treatment in the West. In these studies, patients are divided into two groups: one receives treatment, the other does not. No one—not even the people administering the treatment—knows which group is which. That method works well when studying the effectiveness of medication (one group gets the real thing, the other gets a look-alike placebo, or sugar pill). But it doesn't lend itself to acupuncture studies, since patients and doctors alike know exactly who is getting the needles and who isn't.
- One technique that tries to deal with this dilemma is comparing "real" acupuncture to "sham" acupuncture. In this process, needles are inserted at random rather than at true acupuncture points. The patients don't know if the needles are being inserted at true acupuncture points or not, although the practitioner certainly does. These studies have had mixed results, but most have shown real acupuncture to

be superior to sham acupuncture. The authors note that even when sham acupuncture has been shown to be equally or nearly as effective as real acupuncture, there remains another question: Could it be that needle insertion has some benefit on qi, no matter where the needles go in?

PROBING FOR PROOF

Today the quest for a scientific basis for acupuncture continues. Many researchers in Western countries have now joined in the search. One of the first was Bruce Pomeranz, a neurophysiologist at the University of Toronto who has been studying acupuncture for two decades. His findings have led him to

A Bow to the East

Western medicine recently gave acupuncture a big boost on this side of the Pacific. In March 1996, the Food and Drug Administration (FDA) decreed that acupuncture needles are valid medical tools, not just "investigational" instruments, as previously defined. The FDA stopped short of stating that acupuncture is a proven, effective treatment for various medical conditions. Still, the agency's ruling is expected to bolster the credibility of acupuncture. More people may be willing to try it. And this ruling may bring nearer the day when Medicare, Medicaid, and more private health insurers will cover the costs of acupuncture treatments.

Healing the Pain

believe that acupuncture reduces pain by triggering the nervous system's release of endorphins, the body's naturally occurring painkillers, as well as other substances. Among the latter are ACTH (adrenocorticotropic hormone), a hormone that helps fight inflammation, and prostaglandins, which help wounds to heal.

Although many other research teams have also backed the endorphin theory, it still leaves unanswered questions. For instance: What would explain the other purported health benefits of acupuncture, such as bolstering the immune system or lowering cholesterol levels? The search for more answers is ongoing.

Rather than trying to figure out how acupuncture works, other Western researchers have zeroed in on the question of how well it works. A major area of study has been pain control, which still often befuddles Western doctors.

One of the most comprehensive scientific reviews of acupuncture, appearing in the journal *Pain* in 1986, reported that acupuncture offered short-term relief for 50 to 80 percent of patients suffering acute and chronic pain. Since then, a smattering of studies has appeared in U.S. medical journals. The following are the findings of more recent studies of acupuncture's effectiveness in controlling pain:

• A 1987 study published in *Obstetrics and Gynecology* found that after three months of weekly acupuncture treatments, 10 of

Healing the Pain

11 women with painful menstrual cramps experienced at least a 50 percent reduction in pain. They also used 41 percent less painkilling medication and had fewer headaches, backaches, and other complaints commonly associated with menstruation.

- Researchers at a Danish pain clinic reported in a 1994 issue of the *Journal of Internal Medicine* that acupuncture is a "valuable supplement to the list of migraine prophylactic tools." Acupuncture is especially valuable because it does not induce the fatigue, dizziness, and stomach upset that are common side effects of drugs used for migraine.

- A 1995 study published in the journal *Headache* found that of 26 migraine sufferers, 18 reported at least a one-third drop in headaches after acupuncture treatment. And 15 of them continued to report improved headache relief three years following treatment.

- Patients with painful and inflamed osteoarthritic knees found improvement in their condition after acupuncture treatment, according to an article in a 1995 issue of *Osteoarthritis and Cartilage*.

The newly formed Office of Alternative Medicine within the National Institutes of Health will be funding research on many alternative therapies, including acupuncture. As a result, in coming years we expect to see more scientific evidence of acupuncture's effectiveness.

Healing the Pain

The Big Picture of Chinese Medicine

Many Westerners don't realize that acupuncture is just one element of the overall Chinese approach to health care. Another key aspect of Chinese medicine is the use of herbal remedies, which number in the hundreds. A practitioner usually will combine a regimen of acupuncture treatments along with herbal supplements to be taken in the form of tea, pills, or capsules. In addition, the acupuncturist may recommend dietary and lifestyle changes—all with the goal of achieving a balancing of the meridians.

ACUPUNCTURE'S GROWING POPULARITY

Still, many people are turning to acupuncture to alleviate health problems. The U.S. Food and Drug Administration estimates that roughly 12 million acupuncture treatments are performed each year in the United States. That's an astounding statistic considering that until a quarter century ago, few Americans of non-Asian descent had even heard of acupuncture. Clearly, many people aren't waiting for the scientific evidence.

COMPLICATIONS

The vast majority of acupuncture treatments cause no ill side effects, although some people experience mild nausea or headaches after an initial treatment. Other complications have been reported in the medical literature. Among these are endocarditis (inflammation of part of the heart), hepatitis B and HIV infections, local skin infections, organ injury, pneumothorax (air or gas in the cavity surrounding the lungs), pseudoaneurysm (artery dilation with disruption of artery walls), and spinal cord lesions. These occurrences have been extremely rare, however. As with any invasive medical procedure, the best way to avoid such problems is to see an experienced and well-trained practitioner.

CHOOSING AN ACUPUNCTURIST

Here are a few pointers for guidance if you should decide to see an acupuncturist:

- First, be sure acupuncture is an appropriate treatment for whatever is ailing you. A good acupuncturist will be candid with you about what acupuncture can and cannot do. Some conditions simply don't lend themselves to this form of treatment and instead require conventional medical therapies.
- Check the practitioner's credentials. Not all states have licensing procedures for acupuncturists, and requirements vary greatly among the states that do have them. Learn about the standards in your state. Today both doctors and nondoctors practice acupuncture. Many states don't require M.D.'s to have formal acupuncture training. If you decide to see an M.D. acupuncturist, be sure he or she is a member of the American Academy of Medical Acupuncture, which requires members

Healing the Pain

to have at least 200 hours of acupuncture training. In the case of an acupuncturist who is not a medical doctor, choose one who is certified by the National Certification Commission for Acupuncture and Oriental Medicine, which requires extensive training and testing.

• Ask if the acupuncturist has had experience treating others with the same health problem as yours and if you can speak to those people about their treatment results.

• If you are interested in the entire meridian-balancing approach of Chinese medicine, find out if the acupuncturist uses herbal remedies along with acupuncture treatments. And ask if guidance is offered in dietary and lifestyle changes.

• Ask about needle safety. In this age of AIDS, most acupuncturists use presterilized, disposable needles. Otherwise, the needles should be sterilized in an autoclave (a specially designed apparatus for sterilizing instruments).

• The number of treatments you'll need will depend on your health problem. Acupuncture is not a quick fix. Give it a chance to work. At the same time, if you can't detect any change after a few sessions, you may need to see a different acupuncturist or try another type of therapy.

To find an acupuncturist in your area, get a referral from a friend who's had a health problem similar to yours, consult your physician, call your local and state medical associations, or contact the following:

Healing the Pain

National Certification Commission for Acupuncture and Oriental Medicine

P.O. Box 97075
Washington, D.C. 20090-7075

Send $3 to obtain a list of certified acupuncturists in your state. Or, for $22, you can obtain a complete directory listing acupuncturists and Chinese herbalists throughout the United States and in 20 other countries.

American Academy of Medical Acupuncture

Call 800-521-2262 to request names of physician acupuncturists in your area.

CHAPTER 2
Biofeedback

When you're in pain, you may feel as though you're caught in the unrelenting grip of an uncontrollable force. The more you try not to think about the pain, the more you do. The more you think about it, the more it hurts.

Biofeedback is a technique that aims to break this cycle. It teaches us to modify body functions that we usually consider involuntary—functions such as heart rate, blood flow, brain waves, breathing, body temperature, and digestion. By controlling those functions, we can learn to avoid becoming slaves to our pains and discomforts.

Behavioral approaches such as biofeedback have emerged in an era when more and more people prefer to find nonpharmaceutical methods to manage their pain—or, when possible, to prevent pain altogether. They also want to be actively involved, through self-regulation and self-control, in becoming and staying healthy.

Behavioral medicine, which includes biofeedback training as a subspecialty, is a fairly new branch of modern medical science, dating back only to the late 1970s. Behavioral medicine recognizes that it's not just germs that cause illness; stress, habits, lifestyle, and environment can also be contributing factors.

How Biofeedback Works

In biofeedback, modern electronic equipment is used to monitor internal processes and display them (feed them back) as visual or auditory information. Different devices are used to monitor

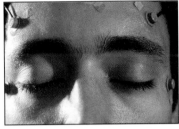

Feedback from an electroencephalogram, which measures brain-wave activity, can help patients learn to relax.

different body functions. For instance, electromyographic feedback devices measure electrical activity in the muscles while thermal biofeedback devices measure skin temperature. Wires run from the instrument to electrodes, or sensors,

that are placed on the skin. There is no pain or discomfort. The biofeedback instrument translates the information it is monitoring into a signal, such as a beep or a blinking light. The patient then learns techniques—such as meditation, deep breathing, relaxation, or visualization—to alter body functions.

Over time, through the process of association, patients gradually learn to link their internal body cues to external biofeedback cues. With practice, they can gain some control over a particular body function, and eventually they no longer need the biofeedback instrument to guide them. At that point, biofeedback techniques can be practiced almost anywhere, at any time. As with any new skill, practice is critical to mastery. The more one practices biofeedback, the more adept one becomes at it.

A Little History

Biofeedback became popular in the United States in the 1960s, a time when many Americans pursued avenues to higher consciousness. The feats of yogis in India, who could control their heart rates, breathing, and other supposedly involuntary body functions, astounded Western observers. Biofeedback was seen as a means to accomplish the same sorts of self-regulatory capabilities without spending a lifetime learning to be a yogi. A decade later, however, biofeedback had become a passing fad. That's when the scientific community started to take serious interest in it. Since 1970, many scientific studies have investigated the alleged merits of biofeedback.

Biofeedback instrumentation has entered new territory in recent years with the advent of computer-based biofeedback. Some therapists believe the computer versions are more informative and motivating for both patients and therapists. By playing a computer video game, patients can learn, for instance, to regulate their heart rate or tame their migraines. Biofeedback instruments can measure a number of different effects, including the following:

- skin temperature, which is influenced by blood flow beneath the skin
- muscle tension, which is measured by an electromyogram (EMG)

Healing the Pain

- heart rate, which is monitored by an electrocardiogram (ECG or EKG)
- galvanic skin response, an indicator of the electrical conductivity of the skin, which is affected by sweating
- brain-wave activity, tracked by an electroencephalogram (EEG)

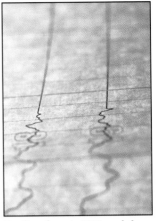

Readings from an EKG can help patients alter their heart rate, which is useful in treating hypertension.

When the body is relaxed, the skin is warm, the heart rate is slow and even, muscles are relaxed, and the mind is alert but at ease. In this state, pain is often reduced and, at times, even eliminated. That is the goal of biofeedback.

BIOFEEDBACK FOR PAIN CONTROL

Biofeedback can help to control the pain or discomfort associated with many conditions, such as:

- anxiety
- back and neck pain
- cancer pain
- fibromyalgia (a migratory muscle-pain syndrome)
- migraines
- muscle injuries
- muscle tension

- Raynaud disease (which involves spasms of the small arterial branches, especially in the fingers and hands and occasionally in other parts of the body)
- temporomandibular joint disorder (TMD)
- tension headaches

In addition to controlling pain, biofeedback has been found useful in treating other disorders, such as asthma, cardiac conditions, dysphagia (difficulty in swallowing), epileptic seizures, fatigue, gastrointestinal problems, high blood pressure, hyperactivity, insomnia, menopausal hot flashes, motion sickness, tinnitus (ringing in the ears), urinary incontinence, and voice disorders.

Multiple studies on the efficacy of biofeedback have appeared in medical publications. The following are summaries of several recent research reports on biofeedback and specific pain-related problems:

Chronic Pain and Disability. Over an eight-year period, researchers studied 354 patients who were judged to be excessively disabled by chronic pain. Their illnesses were diverse and included arthritis, headaches, chronic fatigue syndrome, fibromyalgia, and others. After participating in a six-week behavior management program that included biofeedback, patients showed "significant and lasting reduction of pain and improvement in function at work and at home." One month later, nearly 100 percent of the patients said they would recommend the program; more than 90 percent still said they would recommend it two years later.

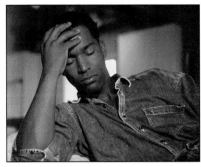
Biofeedback can offer significant relief to those suffering from pain that interferes with daily activities.

Headaches. Research reported in *Psychosomatic Medicine* in 1995 looked at non-drug treatments for headaches in pregnant women. The women who underwent relaxation, skin-warming biofeedback, and physical therapy experienced a 73 percent reduction in headaches. More than half the patients reported significant improvement six months later.

Low Back Pain. In a 1995 study published in *Behaviour Research & Therapy*, patients with chronic low back pain were divided into three groups: those who underwent cognitive behavior therapy, those who practiced biofeedback, and those who were in a control group given no treatment. Both treatment groups had comparable decreases in pain intensity, depression, and disability. However, no such improvements were evident in the control group. A follow-up study six months later showed that both treatment groups had maintained their improvements.

Migraines. A 1995 article in the journal *Headache* reported that migraine sufferers using biofeedback techniques had better

Far-Out Biofeedback

Biofeedback has been used successfully to help NASA astronauts cope with motion sickness, a common ailment in space travel. Antinausea medications aren't effective in space. And while antihistamine injections help, they also make astronauts extremely drowsy. Biofeedback has been found to be a safe, effective alternative. NASA researchers report that about 85 percent of those trained in biofeedback significantly increased their tolerance for motion sickness, and 65 percent managed to suppress their motion sickness completely. Even the 15 percent who didn't show improvement at first did well after additional training.

reduction of pain and less need for medication than those using self-relaxation procedures. Pain in the biofeedback group decreased by 47 percent, and medication usage dropped by 66 percent. Those using self-relaxation experienced decreases of only 14 percent and 1.3 percent, respectively.

GROWING CREDIBILITY

A major breakthrough for the use of biofeedback came in November 1995, when a National Institutes of Health technology assessment panel advocated that behavioral therapies—such as biofeedback, meditation, and hypnosis—be accepted as effective treatment for cancer pain. Panel members recommended that health insurers reimburse behavioral therapies.

Healing the Pain

SIDE EFFECTS

Biofeedback training has no negative side effects. But there is disagreement in the health care community about the effectiveness of biofeedback methods in comparison with other treatments. Some claim that other behavioral therapies, such as hypnosis and progressive relaxation, are superior to biofeedback in controlling pain. A 1995 study in the journal *Pain*, for example, found that training in applied relaxation had stronger short-term benefits for patients with chronic upper-extremity pain than did biofeedback alone or biofeedback combined with relaxation training. After six months had passed, however, the differences between these three treatment groups had vanished.

FINDING A TRAINED PRACTITIONER

Professionals from different health-related disciplines are trained in biofeedback. Your state or local psychological association can provide a list of psychologists who use biofeedback. Or you can obtain a list of trained practitioners in your area by sending a stamped, self-addressed envelope to:

**Association for Applied
Psychophysiology and Biofeedback**

10200 W. 44th Ave.
Suite 304
Wheat Ridge, CO 80033

http://www.aapb.org

CHAPTER 3
Chiropractic

Native Americans, ancient Chinese, the South American Incas, and many other peoples throughout human history have used spinal manipulation of one form or another to combat pain and illness. The first physician to proclaim the benefits of spinal adjustment was Hippocrates, the Father of Medicine himself. He advised his students, "Get knowledge of the spine, for this is the requisite for many diseases."

Today, with some 50,000 active practitioners, the chiropractic profession ranks third in size, after physicians and dentists, among doctoral-level health care providers in the United States. And more people are turning to chiropractors than ever. (Note that although practitioners of chiropractic medicine are sometimes referred to as chiropractic physicians or doctors of chiropractic, in this discussion we only use the term chiropractor to avoid confusion with traditional medical doctors, or physicians.)

In America, chiropractic is the most popular of all alternative therapies, according to a 1990 *New England Journal of Medicine* study. Study results showed that seven percent of the population (or about 18 million people) made an average of 13 chiropractic visits per year, representing a 75-percent increase in use from only a decade earlier. Insurance companies and

Healing the Pain

health maintenance organizations, too, have indicated their support of chiropractic by including it in their benefit plans.

In spite of widespread use and acceptance, there's been a long-running feud between chiropractic and its siblings in the family of health professions. It's no exaggeration to say that the American Medical Association (AMA) waged an all-out war on chiropractic back in the 1960s and 1970s. The AMA formed the Committee on Quackery in 1963, and three years later declared chiropractic an "unscientific cult." The organization even went so far as to advise its members that they'd be guilty of unethical behavior if they associated with chiropractors or referred patients to them.

Chiropractors responded in 1976 by suing the AMA for conspiring to do away with their profession. The wheels of justice turned slowly, but 11 years later the court ruled in favor of the chiropractors. In fact, the court ordered the AMA to reverse its earlier condemnation by stating that it is ethical for physicians to associate with chiropractors in a professional relationship.

Even today, however, many doctors write off chiropractic as quackery. But that's changing. Increasing numbers of physicians acknowledge that there may be something to chiropractic medicine after all, and they know how important nervous-system health is to overall well-being. Many physicians today even refer their patients to a chiropractor for treatment.

Meanwhile, quality research is accumulating to show that chiropractic treatment does help. And although most people associate chiropractic with fixing a bad back, practitioners claim it has achieved excellent results in treating many ailments.

WHAT IS CHIROPRACTIC?

Chiropractic's focus is the spine, which acts as a communications center for the body's nervous system. Because the nervous system connects to every part of the body, chiropractors see it as the key to overall health. Misalignments in the spine—called subluxations by chiropractors—put pressure on the

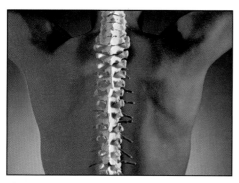

nerves, interfering with normal nerve function. The result: pain and illness. Chiropractors believe that freeing the spine of subluxations, through spinal manipulation or adjustment, will restore health.

Chiropractors view the spine as the key to overall health. Practitioners use several different techniques to adjust the spine and restore health.

Although some people associate chiropractic with body-cracking procedures, many types of chiropractic therapies exist today. A practitioner may use one or a combination of the following:

• A common technique that gently stretches a joint slightly beyond its normal range of motion. Often this causes a

Healing the Pain

Founder of Modern Chiropractic

Daniel David Palmer, a Canadian who later settled in Iowa, is cred-
ited with starting modern-day chiropractic. Palmer had a long-time
interest in natural healing, which he finally pursued professionally.
The healing technique that eventually became known as chiropractic originated one September day in 1895 when a janitor was
explaining to Palmer how he'd lost his hearing 17 years before. He
had exerted himself while in an awkward position and felt something in his back give way. The story piqued Palmer's interest, and
he convinced the janitor to let him try a spinal adjustment. After
three adjustments, the man regained his hearing.

The term *chiropractic* was devised by the Reverend Samuel Weed,
who was one of Palmer's patients. Weed took the term from the
Greek words for "hand" and "practice."

cracking or popping noise, which chiropractors attribute to
a release of gases from joint fluid.

- A gentle-touch technique, which does not involve forceful
adjustment and does not produce cracking sounds.

- A handheld instrument with a rubber tip that gently moves
vertebrae into alignment.

- Network chiropractic, a newer procedure that relies on a specific sequence of adjustments depending on the type and
location of the subluxation.

- Applied kinesiology, a technique based on balancing bones and opposing muscles. Technically, this is not a chiropractic procedure, but some chiropractors use it in conjunction with their other techniques.

In general, there are two broad categories of chiropractic practice: traditional and mixed. Practitioners of traditional chiropractic focus only on spinal manipulation to remove subluxations. Other chiropractors mix several techniques, blending other natural health care therapies such as massage, nutrition and lifestyle counseling, exercise, and heat or cold treatments into their practice.

CONDITIONS HELPED BY CHIROPRACTIC

Most people primarily associate chiropractic with the relief of back pain (especially lower back pain). And that's the use that has been studied the most in clinical research. But practitioners claim chiropractic is helpful in alleviating countless other conditions, too, although little or no scientific research exists to back such claims for many of the conditions. Still, chiropractors report an abundance of anecdotal evidence suggesting that the treatments are helpful. Some of the conditions practitioners say may benefit from chiropractic are:

- aches and pains associated with pregnancy (although special care must be taken in treating pregnant women with spinal manipulation)

Healing the Pain

- allergies
- arthritis
- asthma
- bladder infections
- bursitis
- common cold
- diabetes
- drug addictions
- ear infections
- emotional and mental-health problems
- gastrointestinal disorders
- headaches
- high blood pressure
- menstrual problems
- peripheral joint injuries, such as in the hands, elbows, and shoulders
- poor vision
- respiratory problems
- sexual dysfunction
- sinusitis
- sleep disorders
- sports injuries

Not only do many chiropractors advocate use of their healing techniques to "fix" the body once it's out of balance, they also recommend chiropractic for prevention of health problems.

A well-aligned body, they claim, is better able to stave off disease and dysfunction in the first place.

RESEARCH MOUNTS

Recent research continues to examine chiropractic's credibility as a health care method. These are a few examples:

- A 1992 review by the Rand Corporation of all studies to date on the use of chiropractic for lower back pain concluded: "Spinal manipulation is of short-term benefit in some patients, particularly those with uncomplicated acute low back pain. Data are insufficient concerning the efficacy of spinal manipulation for chronic low back pain."
- The Agency for Health Care Policy and Research acknowledged the short-term value of spinal manipulation for acute low back problems in its 1994 published guidelines.
- A 1995 report published in the *British Medical Journal* compared two groups of patients with low back pain: One group had chiropractic therapy; the other underwent hospital treatment. In all, 741 patients were followed for a period of three years. Based on a questionnaire designed to evaluate elements of back pain, including pain intensity and difficulty in walking, the study found that improvement was approximately 29 percent higher among those receiving chiropractic treatment.
- Looking at chiropractic from the standpoint of cost-effectiveness rather than just patient outcome, a 1996 study

in *Medical Care* found that costs were substantially lower for cases in which chiropractors, rather than doctors, served as initial contact providers.

Even though occurrences of injury due to spinal manipulation are not widespread, episodes have been reported in the medical literature. For instance, a 1995 article in *Neurology* reported on a survey of nearly 500 neurologists, asking them to note neurologic complications in their patients who had been treated with chiropractic. Though the study method was limited, over a two-year period the surveyed specialists reported 55 strokes, 16 myelopathies (diseases of the spinal

Cautions

Sometimes serious health problems—not directly treatable by chiropractic—can manifest themselves as back and neck pain. These include cancer, endometriosis (a condition in which the uterine lining becomes detached and grows in the abdominal cavity outside the uterus), osteoporosis (brittle-bone disease), ulcers, and other organic problems. Your doctor and chiropractor should help you evaluate whether your back or neck pain has origins that are suited to chiropractic adjustment. And they can advise you whether you need another type of medical treatment.

cord or bone marrow), and 30 radiculopathies (damage to the nerve roots entering or leaving the spinal cord). These conditions had developed within 24 hours of a chiropractic visit. Most of the patients had lingering problems three months later, and about half of them experienced severe deficits.

CHOOSING A CHIROPRACTOR

Chiropractors go through an extensive four-year academic program to obtain their doctor of chiropractic, or D.C., degree. Then, before setting up a practice, they must complete a written examination covering multiple topics besides chiropractic per se (anatomy, hygiene, pediatrics, physiology, physiotherapy, X-rays, and more), plus a practical exam that assesses their clinical capability and techniques.

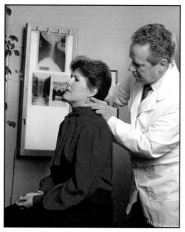

Choosing a chiropractor is like choosing any health care provider. Training, reputation, and personality are all important.

Consider following these recommendations when choosing a chiropractor:

• Get a recommendation from a qualified health care provider. Or ask a trusted friend who's had chiropractic treatment for the same health problem you're experiencing.

Healing the Pain

- Contact your state chiropractic examining board to find out if any disciplinary actions have been filed against a particular practitioner and whether he or she is properly licensed.
- Find out what type of chiropractic therapy is practiced.
- Be wary of anyone who presents chiropractic as a cure for every problem. If the chiropractor tries to talk you out of seeing your doctor or seeking other health care advice, walk away.

Once you've begun treatment

- Remember that overexposure to radiation from X rays can pose health risks, so be alert to the frequency of X-ray procedures, and don't hesitate to ask questions about them.
- If you haven't noticed any change after a few weeks of chiropractic, look into another type of treatment.

FINDING A PRACTITIONER

For additional information on chiropractic and for references to chiropractors in your area, contact your local or state professional chiropractic association. Or contact the major national organization in the United States at the following address:

American Chiropractic Association
1701 Clarendon Boulevard
Arlington, VA 22209
800-986-4636

CHAPTER 4
Cold and Heat
Treatments

Throughout history, humans have used cold and heat to ease pain and discomforts. From Native-American sweat lodges to Scandinavian saunas, people have used heat to relieve tense muscles and stiff joints, as well as to boost general well-being. And cold has been used to treat painful injuries since Hippocrates used ice and snow back in the fourth century B.C. Today, modern medicine still relies on heat and cold to relieve many painful conditions.

USING COLD

There are many forms of cold treatment for pain relief. The most common are ice packs, ice massage, cold compresses, immersion in cold water, or evaporative sprays that leave a cooling after-effect. Commercial ice packs are available, but a bag of crushed ice wrapped in a towel also works well. Refreezable gel packs offer the advantage of being flexible, so they conform better to the shape of the injured area. A bag of frozen peas will do the trick, too.

Whatever you use, be sure there is no direct contact between the ice and the skin. If possible, hold the ice pack in place with an elastic bandage (not too tightly), which will compress the injured area. If you injure a hand or foot, it may be better to immerse it in ice water rather than to apply an ice pack. For an Achilles tendon, put two socks on the injured foot, then stuff a plastic bag filled with crushed ice between the socks to cover the painful area.

ICE FOR MUSCLE AND JOINT INJURIES

Ice is an inexpensive, highly effective treatment for such injuries as sprains, pulled muscles, bruised shoulders, and torn ligaments. Certain types of chronic pain, such as tendinitis and bursitis, also respond to ice treatments. For any of these conditions, ice is most effective when it is applied as soon as possible after the injury or the onset of pain. That's because ice reduces swelling and tissue damage, promoting faster healing. Studies have shown that prompt icing can cut recovery time by as much as half.

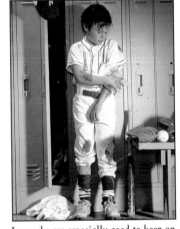

Ice packs are especially good to keep on hand for sports injuries so treatment can begin as soon as possible.

While medical providers agree that immediate icing is crucial, they don't always agree on how long the ice should be applied. It's commonly advised to treat an injured area for

Healing the Pain

RICE for Relief

When you suffer a sprain, strain, pulled muscle, or torn ligament, rely on the RICE routine:

• **R**est to help soothe the pain and to avoid making the injury worse.

• **I**ce the injured area—immediately.

• **C**ompress the injured area to reduce swelling by wrapping it with an elasticized bandage, but be careful not to wrap too tightly.

• **E**levate the injured area to above heart level to help reduce swelling.

10 to 20 minutes. But at least one research group claims that 20 minutes is not long enough, according to a 1995 report in the *American Journal of Sports Medicine*. The University of Chicago research team in this report studied the effect of applying ice wraps to injured knees for 5, 10, 15, 20, and 25 minutes. The 25-minute application did the best job of limiting swelling and internal blood flow, thus enhancing healing. But applying ice for this length of time should probably be limited to the knees or the lower back. Shorter applications of ice are safer for smaller joint areas. An elbow, for example, should be iced for no more than 20 minutes, some experts say, because the nerves are closer to the skin surface. Leaving ice on too long can lead to skin or nerve damage.

After the initial application, apply ice every couple of waking hours (some say more often; ask your doctor) for the next 48 to 72 hours. If swelling or pain returns later, apply ice again.

OTHER WAYS TO USE ICE

Some experts recommend using an ice pack to relieve headache pain. Apply ice either directly to the area where you feel the pain, or place it on the back of your neck. You can also try an ice hat, which is an ice pack that surrounds part of the head.

Many doctors and therapists recommend an ice massage for shinsplints, which are small tears in the muscle attachments on the sides of the shin. The easiest way to do this is to freeze a paper cup filled with water, then peel back the cup's rim so you can rub the ice up and down on your shin muscles from knee to ankle.

Similarly, you can use ice massage for painful heels by rubbing them with a plastic jar filled with ice or by rolling your heels over an ice-filled jar.

CAUTIONS WITH ICE THERAPY

Follow these guidelines to prevent injury from ice therapy:

- Don't put the ice pack directly on your skin. Wrap it in a thin towel to avoid nerve or skin damage.
- Remove the ice for a while when your skin becomes numb.
- Check a refreezable gel pack or chemical ice pack occasionally

for punctures, as the chemicals inside can burn your skin. Be aware, too, that these kinds of packs can be colder than ice, so you may not be able to tolerate them on your skin as long.

- Avoid ice treatment altogether if you're hypersensitive to cold, if you have poor circulation, or if you have any condition that reduces your ability to sense cold.
- Don't put ice directly on open wounds or blisters.
- If you rest while icing, set an alarm or be sure someone is nearby to wake you in case you fall asleep. This will prevent you from inadvertently leaving the ice on too long.
- See your doctor if you fail to see improvement in a day or so.

COLD COMPRESSES

While some experts recommend ice packs for headaches, some people find cold compresses more effective and comfortable. For a tension headache, a cold compress placed against the back of the neck may help. For sinus headaches, apply a cold compress to the forehead and the area below your eyes and above your upper jaw, where sinus cavities are located. Make a cold compress by soaking a cloth in ice water and then wringing it out.

USING HEAT

Heat can alleviate the pain from such conditions as abdominal cramps, arthritis, fibromyalgia, and menstrual cramps. In the case of muscle or joint injury, however, heat is only applied after the injury has been treated with ice for at least 48 hours. Once the swelling is down, heat can be applied to promote healing. At that stage, heat induces greater blood flow, which washes waste products away from the injured area. It also relaxes muscles, prevents spasms, and reduces joint stiffness. If pain or swelling starts to reappear, switch back to ice.

Some doctors recommend foregoing heat treatments altogether. Instead, they suggest alternating icing with moderate exercise sessions. The latter has the same effect of improving blood flow and enhancing healing, and it does so better than heat. Continuing ice applications will keep swelling and pain at bay.

Heat treatments can be dry, such as a heating pad or heat lamp, or moist, such as a hot bath or a hot compress. Both dry and moist heat seem to be about equally effective. Health care providers

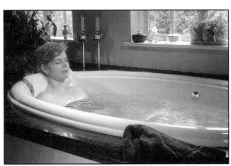

Immersion in a warm bath can help relieve some painful conditions. Applying dry heat, such as a heating pad, can also be effective.

don't all agree on which method is best, but they do agree on one point: Avoid high temperatures. Whether you're applying a heating pad or immersing yourself in a bath, the temperature should feel comfortable to your skin.

In addition to treatments you can do at home, heat treatments are also available through physical therapy or in other medical settings. Whirlpool baths and Hubbard tanks provide immersion therapy. And dipping or immersing a painful joint in paraffin wax can bring relief for such conditions as arthritis. Ultrasound can be used for deeper healing, such as for deep joint pain or fibrous scars. Lasers, microwaves, and shortwaves apply deep heat therapy for pain.

CAUTIONS WITH HEAT THERAPY

- Remember, any external heat treatment should be at a temperature that's comfortable to your skin. Don't overdo it.
- Avoid heat treatments if you have circulatory problems or a condition that impairs your ability to sense heat: The risk of burns may outweigh the advantages of heat therapy.
- Pregnant women need to avoid baths that are too hot. Raising the body temperature above 100 degrees Fahrenheit for a long period could result in miscarriage or birth defects.

HEAT OR COLD—OR BOTH?

For some types of pain, the debate continues as to whether heat or cold is better. For example, heat has been a traditional treatment for low back pain. Yet today many doctors question whether heat is truly the most appropriate treatment for this problem. A research team at the Boston Pain Center studied the use of ice massage, cold pack, and hot pack among patients

Healing the Pain

with chronic low back pain. The researchers found that ice massage was much more effective than the other two treatment methods, according to their report in the 1992 medical textbook *Evaluation and Treatment of Chronic Pain.*

Still, individual preferences must also be considered when making therapy choices. Some back-pain sufferers find ice treatment uncomfortable and prefer heat. After all, a major part of effective therapy is making the patient comfortable enough to continue the process and ultimately to experience relief.

Sometimes therapists recommend alternating hot and cold treatments in what is known as contrast therapy. For example, the Arthritis Foundation recommends soaking hands and feet in warm water (about 110 degrees Fahrenheit) for about three minutes, and then soaking them in cold water (about 65 degrees Fahrenheit) for about a minute. Repeat this sequence three times, then finish with a warm-water soak.

Contrast therapy can be effective for other types of chronic pain as well, such as TMD and tendinitis. A doctor may recommend contrast therapy for a muscle or joint injury—but only after ice has been used long enough to bring down the initial swelling, and the healing process is underway. Nothing but ice, however, should be used for at least the first 48 hours.

Finally, avoid using either heat or cold treatments for gout. Heat increases circulation to the area, and cold may cause more crystals to form in the joint, tendon, or ligament. Either way, you'll end up with more swelling and pain.

CHAPTER 5
Exercise

When some part of your body hurts, your first inclination may be to lie down and not move a muscle. While that can be appropriate when you first suffer an acute injury, it's precisely the wrong thing to do for other pain, such as chronic back pain, headaches, or arthritis. Remaining sedentary in those cases only makes matters worse.

Indeed, the more medical researchers learn about the body's response to pain, the clearer it becomes that exercise is a key factor in pain management. What's more, exercise can often prevent the onset of pain in the first place by improving physical conditioning, which makes us less susceptible to the stresses, strains, and injuries that can result in pain.

EVERYDAY PAINS

At times, even exercise as simple as going for a walk can help prevent or reduce the discomfort of a tension headache. Walking, or any form of physical activity, releases the body's natural painkillers, called endorphins. Activity also relaxes us so we can let go of the day's tensions, which often increase our experience of pain.

Many women have found that exercise brings relief from, and helps them cope with, cramps and other menstrual dis-

Healing the Pain

comforts. For premenstrual symptoms, aerobic exercise may be better than nonaerobic alternatives such as strength training, according to a 1993 study at Duke University Medical Center. Reporting in the *Journal of Psychosomatic Research*, the researchers found that both aerobic and strength-training exercises provided relief for many premenstrual symptoms. But after three months, women

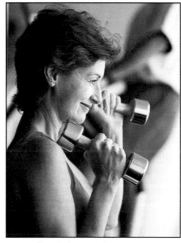

Strength training exercises are recommended for women of all ages to keep the body conditioned, making it less susceptible to strains and injuries.

Warm Up Before You Stretch

Many people assume that stretching before a workout is enough to prevent pulled muscles, tendons, and ligaments. They think of stretching as their warm-up routine. But exercise specialists have learned that stretching cold muscles can also injure them. So it's crucial to warm up for five to 10 minutes **before** you stretch. A warm-up might include a hot bath, walking, light jogging in place, riding a stationary bicycle, or slowly mimicking the movements you'll use in a sport, such as swinging a racket to warm up for tennis.

in the aerobics group showed improvement in more of the symptoms of premenstrual discomfort than women in the nonaerobic group. Improvement was particularly noted with regard to premenstrual depression.

EXERCISES FOR A HEALTHY BACK

Here are a few exercises to do daily to help a bad back get better and then keep it healthy. Remember: Check with your doctor or physical therapist first, especially if you have hurt your back before or you have osteoporosis. After certain kinds of injuries, the following exercises could be bad for you.

Single knee to chest. Lie on your back with your knees bent and your feet on the floor. Grasp the back of one thigh with both hands. Gently and slowly pull it toward your chest until you feel mild tension, but not pain. Hold to a count of ten, without bouncing, then release. Repeat four or five times with the same leg, then switch legs. This exercise stretches muscles in the hips, buttocks, and lower back.

Lumbar rotation. Lie on your back with your knees bent, feet flat on the floor, your arms out to the side for balance, and your heels touching your buttocks. Keeping your knees together and your shoulders on the floor, slowly allow your knees to rotate to the right until you reach a point of mild tension. Hold for a count of ten, then return to the starting position. Repeat four or five times on the right side, then switch to the left.

Healing the Pain

Crunch. Lie on your back with your knees bent, your feet flat on the floor, and your hands gently supporting your head. Slowly curl up just to the point where your shoulders come off the floor. Avoid bending your neck, and exhale as you curl up. Hold for a few counts, then roll slowly back down. Repeat 10 to 15 times to strengthen the abdominal muscles. Strong abdominal muscles reduce the possibility of back injury and help you achieve and maintain good posture.

Chair stretch. Begin by sitting upright in a chair, then bend forward slowly toward the floor. You'll feel a mild stretch in your back. Hold for 15 to 30 seconds; then rise slowly to an upright position again. Repeat the stretch three or four times. This is an easy one to do throughout the day—even at the office—to stretch and strengthen your back muscles.

Cat stretch. Get down on your hands and knees, and while remaining in that position, slowly let your back and abdomen sag toward the floor (sort of like a swayback horse). Hold for a count of five, then slowly arch your back upward toward the ceiling. Hold the position again for a count of five. Repeat this sequence several times.

BACK PAIN

Lying flat on your back is not the best way to cope with chronic back pain. Several studies have shown that exercising to strengthen weak back muscles is crucial for recovery and

Healing the Pain

for the prevention of future back pain. For instance, a study to be published in *Orthopedics* set up an exercise program for nearly 900 people with chronic back pain. They stretched, performed simple back-extension exercises on Nautilus-type machines, and engaged in aerobic exercise, such as riding stationary bikes. Of those who finished the nine-week program, 75 percent reported good or excellent results. A year later, most of the participants said their backs were still in good shape.

If you're currently experiencing back pain, be sure to check with your doctor or physical therapist before starting an exercise program. Once you get the OK, proceed with exercises that don't jar your back or put stress on your spine. Swimming, cycling, cross-country ski machines, and stationary bikes are all good choices. And start your exercise program slowly. If you rush in and overdo it, you risk additional injury.

ARTHRITIS

Arthritis manifests itself in many different forms; two of the most common are rheumatoid arthritis and osteoarthritis. Because joints become stiff and painful, many people with arthritis are tempted to forego unnecessary physical activity. But study after study has concluded that exercise is crucial to keep arthritic joints from becoming stiffer and more painful. For osteoarthritis, research shows that regular exercise can help to improve joint flexibility.

What kind of exercise is best? Research cites benefits from many forms. Because arthritis varies from one individual to the next, it's wise to consult a doctor or physical therapist who can tell you what will work best for your type of arthritis, your type of pain, and your physical ability. Some of the possibilities might include:

- Weight-bearing exercises, such as walking, for strengthening muscles (stronger muscles are better able to support joints)
- Range-of-motion exercises, designed specifically for arthritis sufferers, put the joints through their full extent of movement and help to maintain flexibility
- Stretching, to keep muscles and joints flexible

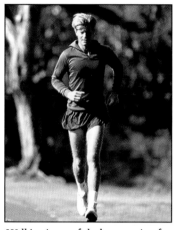

Walking is one of the best exercises for strengthening muscles and building bone.

- Isometrics, in which you create resistance by tightening a muscle without moving the joint, to make the muscle stronger
- Endurance activities, such as swimming and walking, for enhancing aerobic capacity and overall fitness

As a rule, go gently with whatever exercise you do, and always warm up first. Follow the warm up with gentle stretching.

Healing the Pain

Be sure your exercise routine provides a workout for various muscle groups. Start out with a few repetitions; gradually increase the number over several weeks. Some pain and discomfort may occur at first, but don't be discouraged. In time, the dis-

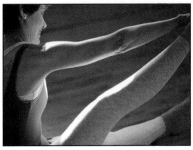

Warm-up exercises and gentle stretching should always precede any exercise program to help prevent injury.

comfort should diminish, and you'll begin to see the benefits. If certain exercises lead to worse or unusual pain, however, stop doing them and check with your doctor or physical therapist.

RANGE-OF-MOTION EXERCISES

Below is a sampling of range-of-motion exercises that can help you live more comfortably with arthritis. Do these exercises gently, without jerking or bouncing. Breathe naturally. If you have any questions about the exercises, ask your doctor or physical therapist.

Thumbs. Open your hand with your fingers straight. Reach your thumb across your palm until it touches the base of the little finger. Stretch your thumb out again and repeat.

Knees. Sit on a chair that's high enough so you can swing your legs. Keep your thigh on the chair and straighten out your knee, but not so that it's locked. Hold for a few seconds.

Then bend your knee as far as possible to return to the starting position. Repeat with the other knee.

Shoulders. Lie on your back and raise one arm over your head. Keep your arm close to your ear and your elbow straight. Return your arm slowly to your side. Repeat with the other arm.

Some therapists have devised creative routines to make range-of-motion exercises less monotonous. For more information about these and other range-of-motion exercises, contact your local chapter of the Arthritis Foundation or write to the national office at 1314 Spring Street, N. W., Atlanta, Georgia 30309.

NECK PAIN

A stiff, sore neck is a common consequence of modern life, the result of too many hours hunched over a desk (or keyboard) or performing repetitive movements. Conditions such as temporomandibular disorders (TMD) and osteoarthritis can also trigger neck pain.

If you have tingling or numbness radiating to your arms or legs, or if your neck pain persists or worsens after three to five days of self care, see your doctor.

For typical neck pain caused by wear and tear on the neck muscles, you can expect considerable relief from the following exercises. Wait to do them, however, until after any acute pain has subsided. These exercises will also help you maintain and

From the East

Many Westerners are discovering the stress-reducing and pain-relieving benefits of exercise methods from across the Pacific.

• *Tai Chi Chuan*, or simply *Tai Chi* (pronounced tie-jee). "Meditation in motion" aptly describes this ancient Chinese exercise. Its slow, gentle movements are reported to be helpful in releasing tension and relieving pain. For instance, *Tai Chi*-based exercises, approved by the Arthritis Foundation, are used to help relieve arthritis pain. And a 1992 study in the *Journal of Psychosomatic Research* reported *Tai Chi* to be as effective in moderating stress as taking a brisk walk.

• *Qigong*, or *Chi Kung*. This is another centuries-old Chinese exercise form, of which *Tai Chi* is one type. Adherents believe that it stimulates and balances the qi (pronounced chee), or life energy, flowing through the acupuncture meridians. Practitioners claim *Qigong* can relieve various physical pains and emotional distresses.

• Yoga. From India, this is another of the world's oldest health practices. Some Western studies have looked at yoga's ability to elevate mood. A 1992 study in *Perceptual and Motor Skills* found yoga to be as helpful as swimming in reducing tension and fatigue. A 1993 British study reported in the *Journal of the Royal Society of Medicine* found that 30 minutes of yoga brought significantly greater increases in mental and physical energy and also in positive mood when compared to relaxation and visualization.

enhance the range of motion in your neck.

Lie down on your back on an exercise mat or a thick carpet. Rest your head on the mat or carpet for support or, if you'd prefer, use a pillow.

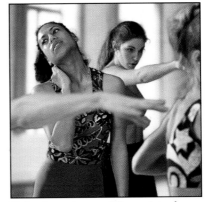

Neck pain can be caused by a variety of activities, including too much time at the computer. A wrong move during exercise class can bring on neck pain, too.

• Move your chin down to your chest and turn toward your shoulder. Hold the position for five seconds. Repeat the movement three times for each side.

• Turn your head sideways as far as possible without discomfort. Hold that position for five seconds. Repeat twice more, then turn to the other side and do the sequence again.

• Move your head to one side so your ear tilts toward your shoulder. Hold for five seconds. Repeat three times for each side.

As you're able, gradually increase the holding times for each of the above exercises from five to ten seconds.

KNEE PAIN

Our knees work hard for us every day, so it's no surprise that some 50 million Americans will have knee pain at some point in their lives. Sprains, runner's knee, and tendinitis are just a few of the conditions that can erupt in pain. Researchers have found that exercising leg muscles is critical to preventing knee problems and alleviating them once they occur.

For example, a 1994 Finnish study published in *Medicine and Science in Sports and Exercise* compared the effects of rest, anti-inflammatory drugs, quadriceps exercise, and other treatments in athletes with knee pain. Exercises were found to be the most helpful in recovery in 70 percent of the athletes.

Here are a couple of exercises to strengthen quadriceps and other leg muscles. (Check with your doctor or physical therapist to be sure these won't aggravate your own knee condition.)

Wall sit. Press your back against a wall; slowly slide downward, keeping your back flat, until your upper legs form a 45 degree angle to the wall. Hold that position for about a minute, tightening the muscles in your buttocks. Your knees should be in line with your feet, not extended beyond them.

Knee extensions. Sit on a sturdy, well-supported tabletop or surface high enough to allow your legs to swing. Attach light weights to your ankles, and grip the surface of the table for balance. Slowly straighten out one leg, but don't lock the knee. Hold for five seconds, then lower slowly. Repeat ten times for each leg.

CHAPTER 6
Herbs

Throughout the ages, herbs have been used all over the world to cure illnesses and heal injuries. Wherever people have lived, they relied on the plant world for substances that would provide relief for illness and injury. Traditional Chinese medicine and East Indian Ayurvedic medicine, for instance, both rely heavily on herbs to treat a vast array of health problems.

But herbal medicine is not an outdated healing regimen. In Europe, for instance, phytomedicine (the medicine of plants) is an integral part of conventional medical practice. Physicians there write prescriptions for herbal medicines, and many are sold over the counter.

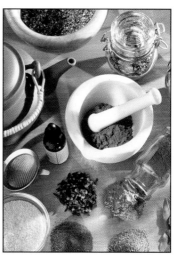

More Americans are turning to herbs, in a variety of different forms, to treat their health problems.

In Germany, students are required to study herbal medicine in medical school, and many insurance companies in Europe cover the cost of herbal remedies.

In the United States today, however, the medical establishment is skeptical about the health benefits of herbs—even though dozens of modern pharmaceuticals are or originally were derived from plants. (Many are now produced synthetically to simulate the plants' effects.) According to a 1985 issue of the *Bulletin of the World Health Organization*, of the 119 pharmaceutical medicines in existence at that time derived from plants, nearly 75 percent were used in modern medicine in ways that paralleled their long-established uses by native cultures as plant medicines. Regardless of their medicinal value, in this country herbs must be marketed as food additives, dietary supplements, or vitamins—not as medicines.

Whether or not herbs are officially designated as medicines, however, more and more Americans are turning to botanicals to treat their health problems. According to herbal industry figures, what was nothing but a fledgling, counterculture industry 20 years ago is now a $1.5-billion-a-year business, with an annual growth rate in sales of 15 percent.

HERBS GET NEW SCRUTINY

The booming popularity of herbal medicine has pushed the medical establishment in the United States to take a second look at it. In early 1995 the Food and Drug Administration (FDA) and the recently formed Office of Alternative Medicine within the National Institutes of Health sponsored a meeting to discuss the potential benefits, as well as the potential problems, posed by the increasing practice of herbal medicine in the United States. At that meeting, both skeptics and proponents of herbal medicine agreed that more research is needed to substantiate the health claims made by herbal practitioners. As with any medical treatment, the FDA wants concrete scientific evidence, not just anecdotal testimonies.

Obstacles exist in producing that kind of research, however. Controlled scientific trials to prove a drug's safety and effectiveness are expensive to run, and unlike conventional pharmaceutical drugs, herbs have no patent protection. Therefore, major drug companies and other research groups have very little financial incentive to pour research and development dollars into studies on herbs.

In addition to the concern that people may not get the health benefits they hope for from herbs, there is the fear that the public may be at risk if the product is unsafe. Regulators would like to see better controls to prevent misidentification of herbs so that buyers are indeed getting what they believe they're getting. Caution is necessary because many consumers have been led to believe herbs are automatically safe because they are "natural" substances. On the contrary, some herbs are toxic and others can be dangerous if used improperly or if contaminated. For instance, according to the 1992 textbook *Adverse Effects of Herbal Drugs*, studies have reported that some Ayurvedic botanical products from Southeast Asia contain extremely high levels of heavy metals. And a report in a 1994 issue of *Lancet* cited a case in which an herbal weight-loss preparation resulted in the deaths of 30 Belgian women due to renal failure. Some of the herbs included in the preparation had been misidentified by the importer, resulting in a toxic combination.

WHAT IS HERBAL MEDICINE?

The herbs used in herbal medicine include plants or plant parts, including leaves, flowers, stems, seeds, roots, fruits, and bark. Some 5,000 different plants are believed to be used for medicinal purposes today.

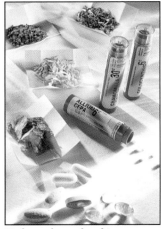

Herbal medicine is believed to work the way any drug does— through the chemicals contained in the plants. Different types of chemicals produce different effects.

Herbs can be purchased in many forms. Dried and encapsulated herbs are perhaps the most familiar.

For example, some boost resistance to stress, some fight disease-causing microbes, some soothe the digestive system, others invigorate the body's metabolism, and so on. But herbs often take longer to work than pharmaceutical medications, especially for more serious health problems. Patience, then, is another essential ingredient in the herbal healing process.

The consumer can find (or prepare) herbs in various forms: fresh, dried, tea bags, capsules, tablets, extracts, tinctures, essential oils, salves, balms, and ointments. Herbs are sold at natural food stores, health food stores, and so-called natural pharmacies; they are also available through mail order. If you feel adventurous you can go it alone, choosing an herb or herbal combination that you believe is suited to your health condition. Or you can take the more prudent approach and work with a health practitioner experienced in herbal therapy. Naturopathic doctors, Chinese medicine practitioners, Ayurvedic doctors, Native-American healers, some conventional doctors, and herbalists all use herbal therapy in working with patients.

Some licensed natural health practitioners, such as naturopathic physicians and traditional Chinese medicine practitioners, have received supervised training in the use of herbs as part of their education. But, in general, no specific license or certification process is required to be a herbalist.

BENEFITS OF HERBS FOR PAIN RELIEF

On the following pages you'll find a list of some painful conditions that are thought to respond to herbal medicine, along with suggestions for remedies. (Note that most of the supporting evidence is based on anecdotal information rather than rigorous scientific analysis.) Prepared herbal products usually come with directions, but you can consult an herbal practitioner for specific information on dosage and frequency for your particular health condition. If you have a serious or chronic health problem, it's wise to seek guidance from a health professional.

Cautions

Under certain circumstances, some herbs should not be taken. Of the herbs mentioned in this section, for example:

• Avoid feverfew if you are taking blood-thinning drugs or if you are pregnant (in fact, don't take any herbal medicines while you're pregnant without first consulting your health practitioner). Some people also get mouth sores and nausea from feverfew.

• Goldenseal must be avoided during pregnancy, as it can trigger uterine contractions.

• Kava kava is contraindicated if you have Parkinson's disease, since it can worsen the condition.

• Chamomile may set off unwanted reactions if you suffer from ragweed allergies.

Arthritis pain. Herbal remedies that are reportedly effective for the relief of arthritis pain include nettles (used topically) or feverfew leaves.

Back pain. White willow bark contains salicin, a natural aspirinlike compound that is claimed to relieve backache symptoms. Cayenne or red chili pepper (available in a cream form) may be useful for lumbago, a dull, aching pain in the lumbar region. Sciatica is said to respond to Saint John's wort when it is taken internally.

Breast pain. Fibrocystic breasts, common among women, feel lumpy and sore. Many natural-health practitioners attribute this condition to improper processing of estrogen by the liver. They recommend a tea made of yellow dock root, dandelion root, burdock root, ginger root, licorice root, vitex, and pau d'arco, which is supposed to stimulate liver function and ease the discomfort of fibrocystic breasts. Bathing in a blend of the essential oils of carrot seed, rosemary, celery, helichrysum, and rose may also be helpful.

Earaches. Garlic in the form of an oil or extract can be administered to the ear to soothe earaches due to infection. Or you can try a few drops of mullein oil, a traditional Native-American remedy for inflammation and swelling. Goldenseal, applied externally or taken internally, may also relieve this type of pain. And echinacea purportedly helps to fight infection by stimulating the immune system.

Menstrual cramps. Herbalists say valerian has a calming effect and that chamomile relieves cramps and promotes menstrual flow. They recommend a mix of ginger, valerian, and cramp-bark tinctures for acute cramps as well as a tea made with fresh ginger root. Or you could try a hot ginger compress (dip a towel in water with ginger essential oil and wring it out) and place it on the abdomen with a hot water bottle over it. This is supposed to increase blood flow and thus relieve cramps. Chasteberry can be tried for painful or irregular menstruation and for premenstrual syndrome. Another potential treatment for multiple menstrual discomforts is made by blending essential oils of chamomile (for anti-inflammation), clary sage (for depression), lavender (a relaxant), and tarragon and marjoram (for cramps). This blend can be massaged into the abdomen.

Migraines. Feverfew leaves have been shown to relieve, and perhaps even prevent, migraines. The Canadian counterpart to the FDA, called the Health Protection Branch, has approved feverfew leaf extract for migraine prevention, provided it contains set minimums of parthenolide, a substance identified as the primary active component in feverfew leaves. Ginger is also recommended for migraines.

Muscle and nerve pain. Peppermint can be used externally. Neuralgia, or nerve pain, may respond to Saint John's wort, taken internally. And leaves from the ginkgo tree are used to treat claudication, a severe calf-muscle pain caused by poor circulation. Chamomile, valerian, cramp bark, and kava kava are thought to relax tense, sore muscles.

Rheumatism. The pain and swelling in and around the joints and muscles may be relieved with nettle or St. John's wort.

Sinus headache. Eating a couple of teaspoons of grated horseradish or sprinkling some cayenne pepper on your food may diminish the pain of sinus headache. You can also mix a small amount of cayenne with lemon juice, honey, and water to make a tea that reportedly loosens mucus secretions and increases blood flow in the sinuses, relieving the congestion that causes sinus headache.

Sore throat. Gargle with a strong sage tea, and you're likely to feel better. A mixture of water and grapefruit-seed extract can also be used as a gargle or drink.

Stomachache. Teas made with ginger, licorice, or peppermint can soothe stomach problems.

Tension headache. Both feverfew leaves and white willow bark are reportedly effective in relieving headaches. Lavender oil can be rubbed into the forehead, temples, and neck to ease nervous tension. Extracts from ginkgo tree leaves are also said to be good for headache pain, as are meadowsweet and skull-cap extracts.

Wounds and bruises. A lotion made with Saint John's wort and applied externally may speed the healing of wounds and bruises. Echinacea or comfrey, used topically, is thought to help the healing of cuts and wounds, but you should never take comfrey internally. Be sure the wound is cleaned thoroughly under running water before applying the herbs. You may also wish to apply a mild antiseptic first. Cayenne powder, mixed into vegetable oil and rubbed into the affected area, is another possible treatment for bruises.

Healing the Pain

FOR MORE INFORMATION...

If you need help finding a qualified herbal practitioner, contact the following:

American Association of Naturopathic Physicians

2366 Eastlake Ave. East, Suite 322
Seattle, WA 98102

Send a check or money order for $5 for a national directory of licensed, accredited naturopathic physicians along with two general brochures on naturopathy.

American Herbalists Guild

P.O. Box 746555
Arvada, CO 80006

National Association for Holistic Aromatherapy

3072 Edison Ct.
Boulder, CO 80301

National Certification Commission for Acupuncture and Oriental Medicine

P.O. Box 97075
Washington, D.C. 20090-7075

Send $3 to get a list of certified acupuncturists and Chinese herbalists in your state, or $22 for a directory covering the United States and 20 other countries.

Healing the Pain

CHAPTER 7
Hypnosis

Most of us have had experiences that provide a glimmer of what it's like to be hypnotized, even if we've never actually been under hypnosis ourselves. Perhaps you've been on a long, boring drive when you suddenly realize that you haven't noticed any of the scenery in the last several miles. Or perhaps you've been so absorbed in a particular activity that you totally shut out all noises and distractions. Very likely, at one time or another, you've simply drifted away for a few minutes, lost in a daydream.

While in the hypnotic state we're neither asleep nor fully awake. We're not conscious, but we're not unconscious, either. The hypnotic state seems to hover somewhere in between, in a sort of twilight zone. Theories abound as to what hypnosis actually is and how it works. But whatever the theory, the experience seems to be that during hypnosis, our normally in-charge conscious mind somehow takes a back seat, while our subconscious comes to the fore. Another way of explaining this, in terms of today's left brain/right brain language, would be to say that hypnosis manages to distract or occupy the left hemisphere of the brain (the logical side) so a person can tap into the resources of the right hemisphere (the intuitive and creative side).

Whichever way we conceptualize the mind, we might think of hypnosis as a tool that helps us relax, focus, and use more of our mind's resources—even those that may lie dormant much of the time. We may become more open to suggestion and to new perspectives. We may be able to see ourselves, our bodies, our feelings, and our abilities in ways that are normally rejected by our purely rational, intellectual side. This is where the therapeutic side—the healing side—of hypnosis comes into play.

HYPNOSIS AND PAIN

Some physicians, psychologists, psychiatrists, natural-health practitioners, and dentists use hypnotherapy (therapy that utilizes the techniques of hypnosis) to help their patients manage their experience of pain—whether it is acute or chronic, whether it is the result of a disease or an injury, and whether the patient is an adult or a child. Pain due to burns, cancer, carpal tunnel syndrome, childbirth, dental problems or procedures, facial neuralgia, menstruation, migraines, osteoarthritis, rheumatoid arthritis, sciatica, tennis elbow, tension headaches, and whiplash, are just some of the conditions that have been reported to respond to hypnosis.

Practitioners also use hypnotherapy to help patients cope with the psychological distresses linked to pain. People in pain often feel anxious, stressed, or depressed, which causes pain to feel worse and triggers a spiraling pain-stress cycle.

History of Hypnosis

Treating ailments by suggestion dates back to early civilizations. Ancient Egyptian priests, for example, used incense and chanting to induce "temple sleep," a trancelike state. Modern hypnosis is traced to Franz Anton Mesmer, a German doctor who practiced what he called animal magnetism in the late 1700s. He was a flamboyant nonestablishment type, and critics were eager to discredit him. Still, mesmerism (as it was called) spread to other parts of the world. Some doctors used it in the days before anesthesia to perform painless major surgery. With the advent of chemical anesthetics, however, mesmerism once again faded away.

It was rescued from oblivion in the mid-1800s by a Scottish physician named James Braid. He came up with the term *hypnosis*, taking it from *hypnos*, the Greek word for sleep. Hypnosis fell in and out of favor repeatedly over the following decades. It was only after World War II that advances in the study of mind and psychiatry renewed an appreciation for hypnosis. By 1958, the British Medical Association had approved hypnotherapy as a valid medical treatment. Three years later, the American Medical Association extended recognition to hypnosis as a therapeutic adjunct, or supplement, to medical treatment.

Scientific research has substantiated claims of pain relief through the use of hypnosis. For instance, a study reported in a 1987 issue of *Kansas Medicine* measured the success of hypnosis in treating 178 people suffering from diverse types of chronic pain, ranging from facial neuralgia, to headaches, to low back pain, to vaginal pain. All participants had been unsuccessful with other pain treatments they had tried. The researchers found that of those patients who later responded to questionnaires, 78 percent were still relieved of their symptoms after six months, 47 percent after one year, 44 percent after two years, and 37 percent after three years.

Several studies completed over the last three decades have found that hypnosis can be helpful to people dealing with cancer pain. One of the more recent studies, reported in a 1992 issue of the journal *Pain*, tested the effectiveness of various psychological techniques for reducing pain in 67 bone marrow transplant patients. To prepare for the transplant, these patients had to undergo extensive chemotherapy, which led to unpleasant and painful side effects such as nausea, oral pain, and vomiting. Researchers found that patients in the hypnosis group experienced less pain of shorter duration than those in the other study groups.

Findings such as these have sparked new backing in the medical community for the use of hypnosis. In late 1995, a technology-assessment panel recommended to the National Institutes of Health that hypnosis and other behavioral therapies be accepted regimens for treating chronic pain. The panel consisted of 12 specialists representing various medical fields; 23 expert consultants presented data to the panel. After reviewing the research to date, the panel found "strong evidence for the use of hypnosis in alleviating pain associated with cancer."

MISCONCEPTIONS PERSIST

Even with the growing acceptance of hypnosis, doubts persist. This is partly due to the side-show image clinical hypnosis has long had to combat. That image has fueled several long-held misconceptions about hypnosis. Some examples follow.

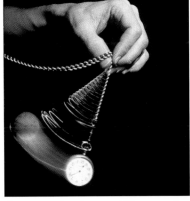

"You are getting sleepy. . . ." For many, the swaying pocketwatch symbolizes their fears about hypnosis.

"The hypnotist will be in control of me." Practitioners point out that the hypnotist's role is to communicate suggestions, using techniques to open the client to accepting those suggestions. Hypnosis is really a relationship of mutual responsiveness, not one in which one person controls the other.

"Only certain types of people can be hypnotized." It is true that some people are more easily hypnotized than others. But even among those who don't respond readily to hypnosis, many can eventually have greater success with it. Sometimes it's simply a matter of moving beyond the fears or negative notions that are blocking receptiveness to hypnosis.

"The hypnotist could make me do something against my will." We've all seen this in the movies: A seemingly normal person is converted into a zombielike machine through hypnosis. While some people may be persuaded to engage in peculiar behavior that they wouldn't allow themselves to do in everyday circumstances, in the hypnotic state they always have control of their actions.

"Once I've been hypnotized, I won't be able to resist it." This is another misconception that revolves around the power issue. The relationship between the hypnotist and the person in the hypnotic state is one of the transfer of power. Many experts on hypnosis see it as enhancing the power of the person under hypnosis.

"I could get stuck in the hypnotic state." Being hypnotized requires the focused attention of the person being hypnotized. The subject can start or stop that state of attention whenever he or she chooses.

"Hypnosis is dangerous." The process of hypnosis itself is not dangerous to your physical or emotional well-being. On the contrary, it can enhance either or both. What could pose risks, however, is working with hypnotists who don't know what they're doing or who are unethical. That's why it's critical to carefully evaluate the credentials of any practitioner you visit (see "Choosing a Hypnotherapist" at the end of this chapter).

SELF-HYPNOSIS

Hypnosis involves focusing attention on certain images, thoughts, or sensations that may have a positive influence on your circumstances—for example, the reduction of pain. You can learn to do these techniques on your own, just as you

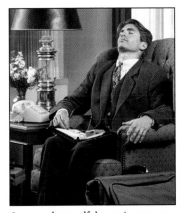

Once you learn self-hypnosis, you can practice it anywhere—a distinct advantage to those who suffer from pain.

might learn some other skill, such as playing a musical instrument. Many practitioners describe all hypnosis as being self-hypnosis, because the subject has to be a willing participant working with the therapist in a mutual relationship.

Hypnotherapists generally teach their patients self-hypnosis techniques, but you can learn

self-hypnosis on your own through books and other resources. An advantage of self-hypnosis is that you have the techniques available to you anywhere, anytime. This is especially useful to someone suffering from pain.

WHAT TO EXPECT

Each person experiences the hypnotic state in a different way. For some, it feels like a state of deep relaxation, with breathing and heart rate slowed and with muscles relaxed. Others feel a heightened sensory awareness or an enhanced

Healing the Pain

Cautions

Neither hypnosis nor self-hypnosis should be used by people who:

• Have epilepsy, since hypnosis might trigger a seizure.

• Are involved in some activity for which they need to be fully alert, such as driving. (Don't be worried, though, that if you're under hypnosis and some unexpected emergency arises, such as a fire, that you won't be able to snap out of it to take needed action. You can always quickly exit the hypnotic state. Still, it's best to not choose to go under hypnosis when you're in the midst of something that requires your full attention.)

• Have serious psychological or emotional problems.

ability to focus attention. Some people say they feel lethargic. Whatever the experience, for most people the hypnotic state is nothing markedly out of the ordinary. Hypnotism doesn't feel magical or mystical.

Some people don't respond to hypnosis at all. Estimates of how many can't be hypnotized vary from one study to another. The World Health Organization estimates that about 90 percent of the population can be hypnotized. Of those, 20 to 30 percent are highly susceptible, entering the hypnotic state quite easily. Most people, if they're willing, can enter the hypnotic state. But that doesn't mean there's something "wrong" with those who can't. There is little agreement as to why some individuals take to hypnosis and some don't. If you decide to try hypnosis, a qualified hypnotherapist would be able to test you for suggestibility.

A key factor in the success of hypnosis is the rapport between the hypnotherapist and subject. Trust and a comfortable environment are crucial elements. If the therapist is unwilling to answer your questions, or if you feel the therapist is trying to foster a dependent relationship, find someone else.

CHOOSING A HYPNOTHERAPIST

Not all states certify hypnotherapists, so be sure to ask about a practitioner's training and experience. For a referral, talk to a trusted friend or your doctor or another qualified health care provider, contact local and state psychological and medical associations, or write to the following national organizations:

American Society of Clinical Hypnosis

2400 East Devon Avenue, Suite 291
Des Plaines, IL 60018

Send a stamped, self-addressed envelope for referrals to doctors and dentists trained in hypnotherapy.

Society for Clinical and Experimental Hypnosis

3905 Vincennes Road, Suite 304
Indianapolis, IN 46268
317-872-7133

Send a stamped, self-addressed envelope to obtain a list of professional hypnotherapists, or request the same by fax at 317-872-7133.

Healing the Pain

CHAPTER 8
Massage

Not that long ago, the mention of massage therapy met with a snicker or roll of the eyes. Many viewed massage as a sleazy activity at worst, a flaky one at best. But in the last couple of decades, attitudes have shifted dramatically. More and more people—of all ages, from all walks of life—are discovering that massage not only feels good, it is good for your health.

Massage is also gaining credibility among traditional medical practitioners; it's even making its way into hospitals and clinics. Its reputation may improve further as published studies emerge from research funded by the Office of Alternative Medicine of the National Institutes of Health. Meanwhile, many doctors, nurses, physical therapists, and massage therapists continue to use massage to alleviate various health problems.

MASSAGE AND PAIN RELIEF

Many types of pain have reportedly responded to massage therapy. These include back pain, cancer pain, carpal tunnel syndrome, fibromyalgia, migraine, muscle strain, neck pain, rheumatoid arthritis, temporomandibular disorder (TMD), tension headache, and whiplash. Massage may also play a role in the prevention of pain. For example, massage can soothe away tension before it triggers a headache, while a post-workout massage may help reduce an athlete's chances of getting sore muscles later on. In addition, massage helps relieve stress, anxiety, and depression, whether these feelings result from illness, injury, trauma, or everyday life's pressures.

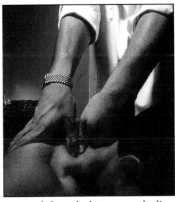

Massage helps to both prevent and relieve pain from a variety of sources, including tension and sore muscles.

How does massage work to relieve pain? One theory is that the pressure from massage closes down the pain gate to the brain, so the pain signals sent by your muscles aren't perceived by your brain. Massage also seems to relax muscular tensions that can trigger pain. And it may improve circulation, reduce stress hormones (such as cortisol and norepinephrine), and stimulate the flow of body chemicals that serve as natural painkillers and mood-elevators. Eventually, research will shed more light on how massage seems to work for pain relief.

A few studies have emerged to support the health claims of massage. Here's what some researchers have reported:

• One study examined the effectiveness of therapeutic massage on pain perception, relaxation levels, and anxiety in cancer patients in a veterans' hospital. All the participants were men, with an average age of about 57. The study involved only two

History of Massage

Humans in diverse cultures have used massage for thousands of years as a means to improve health. The ancient Egyptians treated diseases with massage, and for centuries the Chinese have considered massage to be an essential ingredient of their approach to health care. Hippocrates advocated massage and wrote that "the physician must be experienced in many things, but most assuredly in rubbing."

Modern massage was introduced to the United States in the 1850s by two New York physicians who had studied in Sweden. The first massage therapy clinics were opened here after the Civil War by two men from Sweden. Massage became popular for a while during the 1870s, but public interest in it gradually faded. Today, however, many doctors advocate the value of massage as a useful therapy.

massage sessions, one each on two successive evenings, but the results indicated marked improvements. According to results published in a 1993 issue of *Cancer Nursing*, the men's perception of pain dropped by an average of 60 percent, and anxiety decreased by 24 percent. Feelings of relaxation rose by an average of 58 percent. These subjective evaluations were supported by objective data, which showed decreases in standard indicators of stress, such as heart rate, respiratory rate, and blood pressure.

Healing the Pain

• Researchers at the Touch Research Institute at the University of Miami School of Medicine in Florida looked at the effects of massage therapy on infants and children with various conditions with causes ranging from abuse, to burns, to cancer and rheumatoid arthritis. They found lower levels of anxiety and stress hormones as well as a more rapid recovery among the children, according to their report in a 1995 issue of the *Journal of Developmental and Behavioral Pediatrics*.

A RANGE OF RUBDOWNS

Generally defined, massage is the kneading, stroking, and manipulation of the soft tissues of the body—the skin, muscles,

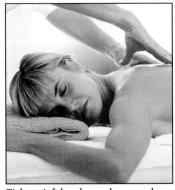

Tight, painful neck muscles respond well to massage therapy.

tendons, and ligaments. But there are dozens of different massage techniques. Some of the more common include:

Swedish massage. Stroking, kneading, and mild tapping of soft tissues are all part of Swedish massage, which is the style most frequently used in the United States. The therapist uses oil or lotion so his or her hands can move smoothly over the skin.

Deep-tissue massage. This technique is similar to Swedish massage, but utilizes deeper pressure to loosen tight muscles.

Healing the Pain

Acupressure. An ancient Chinese technique, acupressure involves various hand and finger movements—pressing, pushing, rubbing, squeezing, and the like—on designated areas (acupoints) along the body's meridians, or energy pathways. The purpose of acupressure is to open blocked energy channels that result in disease or pain. See the chapter on acupuncture for the philosophy behind this method.

Shiatsu. This is a Japanese version of acupressure.

Reflexology. Reflexology is massage that focuses on the feet and sometimes the hands. Specific points on the feet and hands are thought to correspond to parts of the body, including the glands and organs. The therapist applies pressure to these points for diagnostic purposes and to stimulate healing of the related body part. Many doctors have reservations as to the validity of this type of massage, however.

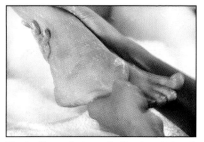

The healing technique of reflexology is based on principles similar to acupuncture.

Sports massage. Specifically tailored for the athlete, sports massage focuses on parts of the body that get frequent use in a particular sport. For example, the legs of a cyclist and the arms of a swimmer get special attention. Massage before athletic activity helps warm up the muscles, while a post-workout

Cautions

Massage should never be applied to the site of an open wound, injury, cancer, or skin infection. People with a history of blood clots should avoid deep, high-pressure massage techniques that might loosen a blood clot and cause an embolism. If you have any doubts about whether you have a health condition that would contraindicate massage therapy, talk to your doctor first.

massage seems to stimulate blood circulation and clear away lactic acid residues that cause muscle soreness.

Trigger-point therapy (also called myotherapy). Trigger points are sensitive spots in the muscles that are often painful. They result from repetitive motions, injuries, accidents, or other trauma. Over time, disease and aging can increase the painfulness of these points. Deep pressure applied to these areas can relieve pain. For chronically irritable trigger points, several sessions may be needed to completely clear the problem.

FINDING A MASSAGE THERAPIST

To locate a massage therapist in your area, contact:

American Massage Therapy Association
820 Davis Street, Suite 100
Evanston, IL 60201

CHAPTER 9
Nerve Blocks

The nerve block is a century-old technique for evaluating and treating pain. A chemical agent is injected on or near a particular nerve to block the transmission of painful stimuli along the nociceptive pathways (pathways that transmit pain signals triggered by physical or chemical damage in the body's tissues). Although *nerve block* is used in the singular, there are many types of nerve blocks.

While modern medicine is devoting increasing attention to the psychological aspects of pain, many medical specialists feel nerve-block techniques are a valuable component of a pain-management program. What's more, nerve blocks may help to make other forms of therapy possible. For example, with a nerve block it may be possible to leave motor ability intact but selectively block out painful sensations, so a patient would be able to undergo physical therapy and exercise even while suffering from a painful musculoskeletal condition.

Overall, nerve blocks fall into two broad categories:

- Neurolytic blocks use injections of substances such as phenol or alcohol, which result in destruction of the nociceptive pathways. But neurolytic blocks rarely relieve pain permanently, and repeated treatments may be needed. In addition, side effects can be profound and might include damage to neighboring nerves and loss of muscle function. Therefore, neurolytic blocks are usually reserved for severely ill patients with a limited life expectancy.

• Nonneurolytic blocks use injections of nondestructive substances, usually including local anesthetics such as lidocaine or bupivacaine. Sometimes the injected substance is a combination of local anesthetics and other agents, such as corticosteroids. Nonneurolytic blocks impede pain transmission without destroying the nociceptive pathways, giving them a wider range of therapeutic uses.

Nerve blocks are invasive procedures for pain relief and are somewhat painful and stressful in themselves. The patient is usually given a local anesthetic to anesthetize the area in preparation for receiving the nerve block. The doctor's skill and experience are crucial ingredients in the success of these procedures. In most cases, the administering physician will be an anesthesiologist. Whoever performs the nerve block should be familiar with managing toxic reactions to local anesthetics and with resuscitation techniques. The administering physician should also have emergency resuscitation equipment on hand in case the patient experiences an adverse reaction to the nerve block. Sometimes patients receive nerve blocks on an outpatient basis; in other cases, brief hospitalization is required.

Healing the Pain

FUNCTIONS OF NERVE BLOCKS

Nerve blocks can be effective for treating both acute and chronic pain. Acute pain is usually intense but of short duration and is brought on by injury, surgery, or other trauma. In contrast, chronic pain persists over a long period of time. In pain treatment programs, nerve blocks can serve various functions as described below:

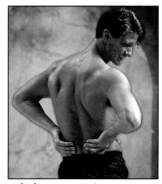

Whether your pain is acute or chronic, nerve blocks can bring relief. They can also be effective tools in the diagnosis of painful conditions.

Diagnosis. Nerve blocks may help doctors identify the site and cause of pain. For example, a nerve block can distinguish between local pain (pain at the site at which it is sensed) and referred pain (pain caused by a problem in some other part of the body). Doctors can also administer nerve blocks in order to get a picture of a patient's condition in the absence of pain. How does the patient's behavior change? What physical limitations exist, if any, that are unrelated to the pain the patient feels?

Prognosis. A prognostic nerve block helps physicians predict the outcome of other procedures that would permanently block a nerve. For example, for certain types of pain, doctors might consider surgery on the nervous system or an injection that would permanently block transmission of pain in a specific area of the body. Using a nerve block can simulate, at least to some degree, the result of these types of permanent or long-term procedures and, therefore, help the physician to evaluate their effectiveness.

Prophylaxis. In the medical literature, some evidence that nerve blocks can prevent pain from developing has begun to emerge. Administering a nerve block before certain types of surgeries may ward off some postoperative pain syndromes. The research on this procedure is still inconclusive, however.

Therapy. Besides dealing with the site and source of the pain itself, nerve blocks can help in other ways. For instance, somone in pain may develop muscular tensions and postural abnormalities that set off more spasms and immobility—and then more pain. A nerve block can interrupt that cycle. Still, contrary to the hopes or expectations of many patients, permanent pain relief usually doesn't result from a one-time nerve-block injection. Pain relief may last for periods ranging from hours to weeks or months, depending on many factors. To get long-term pain relief, additional treatment may be necessary along with ongoing nerve-block therapy.

Many nerve-block specialists combine blocks (for immediate pain relief) with treatments such as physical therapy or other rehabilitation. These procedures may be more effective when used together, leading to better and faster pain relief.

CONDITIONS BENEFITED BY NERVE BLOCKS

The following is a summary of various types of pain that may be alleviated by a nerve block:

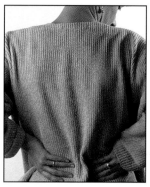

Nerve blocks are often used to treat severe lower back pain.

Nerve pain from spine problems. The most common block for this type of pain is an epidural block or injection, which usually includes a local anesthetic and an anti-inflammatory steroid medication. The purpose is not only to provide pain relief, but to allow for rehabilitation or physical therapy, as well.

Cancer pain. When pain medications and therapies don't work to relieve cancer pain, nerve blocks may be helpful. Neurolytic blocks have proven especially helpful in treating pain from cancers affecting inner organs in the trunk and torso. For instance, various studies have reported success rates of 70 to 80 percent in bringing immediate relief to patients suffering from pancreatic cancer. Pain symptoms from other forms of upper-abdominal cancer, pelvic-organ cancer, and cancer of the head and neck respond well to nerve blocks.

Myofascial pain syndrome. This type of pain is usually steady, deep, and aching. It's centered around various hypersensitive points in the muscles called trigger points. When irritated,

Healing the Pain

these trigger points set off referred pain (pain felt somewhere away from the trigger point) or local pain. If left untreated, myofascial pain syndrome can become chronic and debilitating. Local anesthetic injections at trigger points act like nerve blocks and bring relief from painful symptoms. Effective treatment must also aim to correct the cause of the irritation of the trigger points.

Peripheral vascular disease. This is a broad medical category for circulatory problems that affect the body's extremities. Among such conditions are Raynaud disease, which involves spasms of the small artery branches (especially in the fingers and hands) and frostbite. When these conditions are severe, a nerve block might be considered for pain relief.

When to Rule Out Nerve Blocks

Nerve blocks usually are not advised when:

• the patient has a blood-coagulation (clotting) deficiency

• an infection is present, particularly if it is in the area of the nerve-block injection site

• the patient has a low stress or pain tolerance

• the patient is unable to fully cooperate for some reason—perhaps due to a language barrier or an inability to understand the procedure.

Healing the Pain

Reflex sympathetic dystrophy (RSD). This painful condition may result from various physical traumas, ranging from a fracture to surgery to a stroke. But RSD can also show up without any evidence of physical trauma, making it more difficult to diagnose and treat. Nerve blocks have proved to be useful diagnostic and therapeutic tools for RSD. Treatment might involve repeated nerve-block procedures over a period of time or a continuous block, provided by means of an indwelling catheter. Nerve blocks are most effective in RSD if started within three to six months of the onset of symptoms.

Shingles and postherpetic neuralgia. Also known as herpes zoster, shingles is a painful viral infection of one or more nerves that produces a blistery, itchy skin rash. After the rash has disappeared, patients may experience postherpetic neuralgia, a painful condition that persists for months, even years. Several studies have shown nerve blocks to be highly effective for treating shingles—if used in early stages of the disease.

Other types of head and neck pain. Severe migraines, cluster headaches, and tension headaches that fail to respond to less invasive therapies can sometimes be successfully treated with nerve blocks, as can pain from whiplash or facial neuralgias.

ADVERSE EFFECTS

Any type of nerve block can cause bleeding, infection, and accidental puncture of organs, arteries, or other body structures near the injection site. Neurolytic blocks have the added risk of causing unplanned permanent neurologic injury—such as paralysis, sensory loss, or painful neuralgia—if the neurolytic solution somehow spreads into other nerves near the target nerve. For that reason, many pain-management specialists feel that neurolytic blocks should be performed under the guidance of fluoroscopy (a procedure that displays images on a televisionlike screen) or computed tomography (a system that uses successive X rays taken at slightly different angles to create a three-dimensional image).

In addition to the complications already mentioned, each of the many different nerve block procedures has other potential side-effects, some minor, others serious, and a few even life-threatening. A doctor performing a nerve block should fully inform the patient beforehand about what to expect in terms of pain relief and adverse reactions.

CHAPTER 10
Over-the-Counter Medications

Not that long ago, over-the-counter (OTC) pain relief medication meant one thing: aspirin. It's not so simple anymore. These days some 200 different versions of nonprescription pain relievers line the shelves at your local pharmacy. The sheer number is overwhelming, but so are the claims, each one declaring that it provides faster relief, longer-lasting relief, relief without upsetting your stomach, and more.

Faced with this marketing deluge, you need to be smart when choosing and using over-the-counter pain medications. You need to ask: Do some work best for certain types of pain? What risks, if any, do I run by using these products? How do I minimize those risks for myself and my family?

OTC CATEGORIES

The two broadest categories of OTC medications for pain relief are NSAIDs (nonsteroidal anti-inflammatory drugs) and acetaminophen. Aspirin, the first NSAID to become available over

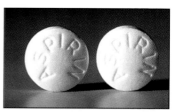

Aspirin was used for pain relief long before other over-the-counter NSAIDs.

Brand Name vs. Generic

What's the difference between brand-name OTC pain relievers and generics? Mostly, it's price. Generics almost always cost less. And contrary to what many people believe, generic products are just as effective as their brand-name counterparts. That's because they contain the same active drug, although they may include different types or amounts of inactive ingredients.

the counter, has been a household pain reliever for nearly a century. Ibuprofen, the next NSAID to become available without a prescription, was approved for OTC sale in 1984. (It first appeared a decade earlier as a prescription medication.) By 1996, two additional NSAIDs had come out as OTCs: naproxen sodium and ketoprofen. Acetaminophen, which is not an NSAID, made its debut as a nonprescription drug in the mid-1970s. New OTCs are likely to become available in the near future.

All OTC NSAID medications work with about equal effectiveness to relieve minor aches and pains, such as backache, headache, menstrual cramps, sore muscles, and toothache. But some are more effective for specific types of pain, and others just seem to work better for certain people. Potential side effects are generally similar, but vary somewhat among individuals. All these factors have a bearing on which OTC pain reliever is right for you. In the following sections we'll look more closely at each medication.

ACETAMINOPHEN

Acetaminophen, known by such brand names as Tylenol, Pamprin, and Excedrin, is also available in generic form. It relieves the pain of headaches and sore muscles, and it reduces fever. Unlike the NSAIDs, however, acetaminophen does not reduce inflammation. This makes it of limited use for pain caused by rheumatoid arthritis and other inflammatory conditions. But it has proved effective for osteoarthritis, which does not usually involve inflammation. No one knows for sure how acetaminophen works, but some theorize that it may act on nerve endings to suppress pain.

BENEFITS OF ACETAMINOPHEN

Some of the key benefits of acetaminophen over other pain relievers include:

- It's least likely to cause stomach and gastrointestinal problems.
- It can be used by people who have allergies to aspirin and those who have ulcers.
- It doesn't reduce blood clotting, so it is useful for people who are taking blood-thinning drugs.

Because of these benefits, many experts view acetaminophen as the safest of the OTC pain relievers.

RISKS OF ACETAMINOPHEN

Excessive doses of acetaminophen have proved to be toxic to the liver, and alcohol further enhances the toxic effects of high doses. Some researchers contend, however, that even smaller doses of acetaminophen may be toxic to the liver for people who regularly use alcohol. For example, a study reported in a 1995 issue of *Hepatology* looked at 67 regular users of alcohol who had liver damage linked to acetaminophen usage. They had taken the medication for periods ranging from one day to several months. Most of the study's subjects were alcoholics or heavy drinkers, and many took overdoses of acetaminophen.

But not all subjects who had liver damage had misused the acetaminophen or overindulged in alcohol. Forty percent had taken the recommended dosage of the medication, and 35 percent had had three or fewer drinks per day. Actually, the incidence of liver toxicity among people who drink and take acetaminophen is extremely low considering how many people do both. Still, the study raises the question: Could some people be especially susceptible to this type of liver damage?

Alcohol use may not be the only cause for concern among those who use acetaminophen. Liver toxicity has also been reported among people on acetaminophen who are fasting or just not eating properly (perhaps because they're ill and don't feel like taking in food). A study published in a 1994 issue of the *Journal of the American Medical Association* found that a daily dosage of between four grams (the maximum recommended daily dosage for adults) and ten grams put fasters at risk for liver toxicity.

The upshot of these studies is that you may hear divergent advice about how to use acetaminophen safely. Some doctors feel that adhering to recommended dosages is enough to protect you. Others advise that anyone who drinks three or more alcoholic beverages a day should cut acetaminophen intake by half. Additional studies will be required to supply more definitive information on the connection between acetaminophen use and fasting and/or drinking alcohol.

In the meantime, the Food and Drug Administration now requires all pain relievers that attained OTC status after 1994 to carry this warning: "If you generally consume three or more alcohol-containing drinks per day, you should consult your physician for advice on when and how you should take [product name] and other pain relievers." Manufacturers of other OTC pain relievers have been asked to include this warning voluntarily, and some have already done so.

Research has also found that heavy use of acetaminophen may be related to kidney problems. More than 700 patients with kidney failure were interviewed about their own past use of pain-relieving medication. Their responses were compared with those of more than 300 other people without kidney disease. The results, published in the *New England Journal of Medicine* in 1994, showed that people were twice as likely to have kidney

OTCs Plus Caffeine

Some manufacturers add caffeine to pain relievers, claiming that it boosts the effects. The research on this subject is fairly thin, however. Caffeine may enhance pain relief by lifting a person's mood, but you could get the same result by taking the OTCs with a cup of coffee. Bear in mind that some pain problems (particularly headaches) may be worsened by caffeine, and if you take caffeine-fortified OTCs at bedtime, you may set yourself up for a sleepless night.

failure if they'd taken more than one acetaminophen pill every day for a year (labeled as "heavy" usage) or if they'd taken 1,000 or more pills in their lifetimes (considered to be "medium-to-high" cumulative intake).

NSAIDs

All the nonsteroidal anti-inflammatory drugs, or NSAIDs, relieve pain by blocking the body's production of prostaglandins. Prostaglandins are hormonelike chemicals that—among many other functions—can send pain signals to the brain and cause inflammation. NSAIDs not only relieve headaches and other everyday pains, they also ease the pain and swelling of arthritic diseases and sprained muscles.

The *nonsteroidal* part of their name sets NSAIDs apart from corticosteroids, which also block prostaglandin production but

Healing the Pain

have more dangerous side effects. Long-term exposure to corticosteroids can cause many problems, including cataracts, diabetes mellitus, high blood pressure, immune-system impairment, osteoporosis, and severe mental disturbances. NSAIDs, in contrast, pose fewer of these risks.

Benefits of NSAIDs

Of the four NSAIDs available over-the-counter today, aspirin (or acetylsalicylic acid) is the old-timer. It's still a popular medication for many common, everyday pains.

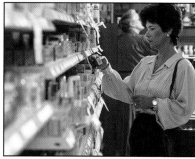

As for the other three NSAIDs—ibuprofen (Advil, Motrin-IB, and Nuprin), naproxen sodium (Aleve), and ketoprofen (Actron and Orudis KT)—all are equally effective for pain, according to statistical data. These are especially useful for menstrual cramps, toothaches, minor arthritis, and injuries characterized by inflammation, such as tendinitis. Choosing one of these medications over another is often simply a matter of personal preference. No clear-cut, published clinical research shows any of the three to be superior for a particular pain condition. Still, one person may experience better results, with fewer side effects, from one NSAID than another.

Personal preference often dictates the choice of over-the-counter pain relievers, as none of the NSAIDs has been proved most effective.

Risks of NSAIDs

High doses of NSAIDs can cause stomach pain as well as serious gastrointestinal bleeding, ulceration, and perforation. The latter serious side effects occur infrequently—in about one to two percent of patients—but they can hit suddenly, without warning symptoms. Each year about 76,000 people in the United States end up in the hospital due to NSAID-related stomach problems, and about 7,600 people die each year from these problems. People at highest risk include those who take high doses for prolonged periods, such as those who suffer from arthritis and other chronic pain conditions.

As is true of acetaminophen, NSAIDs have been linked to kidney failure, according to the 1994 *New England Journal of Medicine* study mentioned previously. People who had taken more than 5,000 NSAID pills in their lifetime (considered a "high" lifetime intake) were four times more likely to have kidney failure than those who took less than 1,000 pills. Interestingly, aspirin is the exception here; its usage was not correlated with increased risk of kidney failure.

But aspirin carries the other risks of NSAIDs already mentioned, plus a few more:

• Children and teenagers with chicken pox or the flu should never be given aspirin because it may lead to Reye syndrome, a rare disorder that can cause seizures, brain damage, and even death.

Healing the Pain

- Anyone with gout should avoid all salicylates (including aspirin) because these medications may increase the number of attacks of gout.
- Some people are allergic to aspirin. Anyone with an aspirin allergy should avoid taking it, products that contain aspirin, and any other NSAIDs.
- Some people with asthma find that aspirin can trigger an asthmatic attack (this is also true for other NSAIDs).
- Aspirin should not be taken by people with bleeding disorders or who are taking anticoagulant medication unless they are carefully monitored by their physician. (This also applies to other NSAIDs.)
- Women in their last trimester of pregnancy should not use aspirin because of the risk to the fetus as well as the risk of maternal and fetal bleeding during delivery.
- People with uncontrolled high blood pressure who take aspirin run the risk of having a stroke. On the other hand, when high blood pressure is controlled and the use of aspirin properly monitored, aspirin can help reduce the risk of stroke.

As for relatively minor side effects, NSAIDs can make you dizzy, anxious, drowsy, or confused. Aspirin and some NSAIDs have been known to cause tinnitus, a ringing or buzzing in the ears, but this usually disappears when you stop taking the medication.

Healing the Pain

What Does All This Mean?

The pros and cons of taking OTC medications for pain are confusing. There is no simple, one-size-fits-all answer to the question of whether or not you should take them. Keep in mind that people with certain health conditions are more vulnerable than others to serious side effects; they need to exercise extra caution.

Most medical experts believe that OTC pain medications are helpful, not harmful, for most people if used properly. That means taking a medication occasionally, when you really need pain relief. Popping pills every day, for weeks or months on end, is reckless and asking for trouble. We too easily forget that OTCs are potent medicine—even if they're nonprescription.

Here are a few guidelines on using OTCs:

Read the label. You hear this all the time, but most of us never do it. It's a hassle, the print's too small . . . excuses abound. But it is important to know what you're taking, whether it's the right medication for the type of pain you have, and how to use it. You may also see extra cautions for usage by children or the elderly.

Once you've read the directions, follow them carefully. If one pill will take care of the pain, many people figure two (or three) will zap it faster, better. This "more is better" mentality is dangerous. Take no more than the recommended dosage at the specified time intervals.

Avoid prolonged use. No OTC is meant to be used for a long period of time without a doctor's supervision. If pain persists, you need to find and treat the cause. See your doctor if symptoms last longer than ten days.

Still More Choices

Not only do you face a selection of types of pain relief compounds, but each type also has variations galore. Here's a little help in sorting out product descriptions:

Enteric-coated: These products have a coating so the pill will pass through the stomach and not dissolve until it reaches the small intestine. This lessens the chances of getting ulcers and stomach irritation, but it does not eliminate those concerns. And because coated pills dissolve more slowly than uncoated ones, pain relief is delayed.

Extra-strength: Use this type when you find yourself needing more than one regular-strength pill to relieve your pain.

Timed-release: These products dissolve slowly, with the result that a more constant level of pain reliever is maintained. Use timed-release medication when you need lasting, but not immediate, relief.

Buffered: These pills contain an antacid to reduce the risk of stomach problems. Experts don't agree on whether this works. Those who believe it works also disagree on how effective it is.

Watch your medication mixtures. Some European studies have shown that mixing different types of painkillers, such as NSAIDs and acetaminophen, and taking them for a long period of time, may increase the chances of kidney damage. That concerns many experts, including the National Kidney Foundation, especially in light of the rising rate of kidney failure in the United States. Although studies to date are inconclusive, you're probably better off taking one kind of OTC pain reliever at a time. And when your doctor gives you a prescription, tell him or her what OTCs you're currently taking so you don't get negative interactions or counteractions between the two types of medication.

Questions. Finally, if you have any doubts about using an OTC pain reliever, talk to your doctor or pharmacist. Knowing your medical condition and the reason you're seeking pain relief, they can best advise you about the pros and cons of taking any of the OTC pain medications. It's always better to consult a professional first.

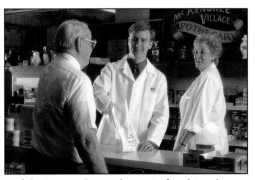

Don't hesitate to ask your pharmacist for advice when choosing an OTC pain reliever. The pharmacist can explain which OTC may be more effective for your pain.

CHAPTER 11
Pain Clinics

Living with pain used to mean "toughing it out." Today, however, *living with pain* means learning how to cope and how to keep pain from controlling you, so you can get on with your life.

That transformation has come with a change in modern medicine's approach to pain. Health professionals now view pain as a major public health problem, not just an inevitable accompaniment to illness and injury. Now more than ever, researchers are scrutinizing pain, trying to understand how it works, and experimenting with ways to counteract it. In addition, a variety of pain clinics (also called pain centers) have been established that are devoted to the evaluation and treatment of pain. By the early 1990s, an estimated 2,000 pain clinics existed in the United States.

Although these facilities differ in staff makeup, size, and their approach to pain treatment, most pain clinics focus on patients with chronic pain. Unlike acute pain, which eventually disappears, chronic pain lingers and feels as if it will never go away. Chronic pain might result from injury or disease, or it may seem to come out of nowhere, untraceable to any specific cause. It can range from mild to excruciating. Whatever the source or degree of discomfort, there's one common element in chronic pain conditions: It changes people's behavior. The relentlessness of the pain wears them down physically and emotionally, can make them feel helpless, and may even lead to clinical depression (a severe form of depression). People who suffer from chronic pain are the ones referred to pain clinics by their doctors. By the time they get there, they have usually run the gamut of doctor visits, tests, retests, and treatments, yet their pain persists. For people suffering from chronic pain, dealing with that pain has become the focal point of their lives.

TYPES OF PAIN CLINICS

The term *pain clinic* has come to apply to many different types of facilities, ranging from the small one-doctor operation that treats only one kind of pain to the clinic that's staffed by many different health professionals offering diverse treatments. To clarify what constitutes a pain clinic, the International Association for the Study of Pain (ISAP) in 1991 set down a classification system dividing pain facilities into four categories:

Modality-oriented clinic. This type of pain clinic furnishes one or only a few types of treatment for pain. For instance, it may concentrate only on nerve blocks or biofeedback training.

Pain clinic. This facility provides diagnosis and treatment of chronic pain, perhaps specializing in one part of the body. But these clinics do not provide as comprehensive an assessment and treatment as the two types of facilities listed below.

Healing the Pain

Multidisciplinary pain clinic. Clinics in this category specialize in the diagnosis and treatment of chronic pain through a combination of health care specialties, such as anesthesiology, psychology, and physical therapy. Patients can be treated on an inpatient or outpatient basis, or both, depending on their particular needs.

Multidisciplinary pain center. This is much the same as the multidisciplinary pain clinic, but it also does pain research. These centers typically are connected to a medical school or teaching hospital. They may offer both inpatient and outpatient treatment programs.

WHAT TO EXPECT AT A PAIN CLINIC

Of the four categories of pain clinics described above, the multidisciplinary types are the ones pain experts most often recommend for people with chronic pain. Still, not everyone with chronic pain needs a multidisciplinary facility. But for the patient with a more complex set of problems who has tried many options with no success, a multidisciplinary clinic or center may be the best next step.

The multidisciplinary approach uses many different types of health care expertise to diagnose and treat a person's pain. Each individual's pain is different, so the treatment technique that works well for one person may not work as well for another, even for the same painful condition. The staff works together to assess the pain problem and then designs a treatment plan especially for that specific individual.

The staff at a multidisciplinary clinic or center might be made up of dentists, physicians, nurses, nutritionists, occupational therapists, pharmacists, physical therapists, psychologists, social workers, vocational rehabilitation counselors, and other health care providers. Multidisciplinary centers also have research staff who may specialize in various fields. The full-time facility director will be a specialist in one of these disciplines, but should also be a believer in the comprehensive approach to pain treatment.

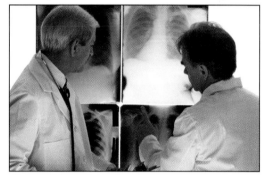

Doctors on staff at a pain clinic study X rays to help evaluate the patient's problem. After examining the patient and reviewing tests, they will recommend a treatment program.

All of the staff members combine their expertise to assess the particular pain problem. They'll ask about the patient's pain complaints, try to trace how the pain started, and look at other aspects of the medical history. They'll review test results done elsewhere and undertake further evaluations if needed.

Once they determine the sources of pain and how these factors affect the patient's life, they'll design a treatment plan. Treatment approaches may include many of the techniques described in detail in other chapters in this book. Most clinics will use several treatments, ranging from the more conventional, such as counseling, physical therapy, and transcutaneous electrical nerve stimulation (TENS), to the less conventional, such as acupuncture, hypnosis, and meditation. Each patient's program is designed to help that person learn ways to manage the physical, psychological, and emotional components of his or her pain.

The treatment team will want to work not only with the patient, but also with family members and, perhaps, the patient's employer. After all, they, too, are living with the patient's pain and can help or hinder progress, often unknowingly. For instance, if they're overcritical they might sabotage whatever progress has been achieved through treatment. But they can inflict just as much damage by being too sympathetic and overly attentive to the patient's moods and complaints. Thus, chances for successful treatment are best if the whole family knows what to expect and what to do.

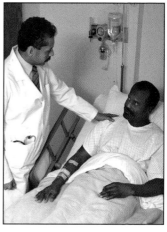

Pain clinic programs may be based on inpatient or outpatient treatment. Sometimes a patient will stay at the clinic for a few days, occasionally even for a few

Whether a patient is treated on an inpatient or outpatient basis depends on the clinic and the treatment program.

weeks. At other times the patient may come in for regular treatment as an outpatient. One clinic may offer either type of arrangement, or both, depending on what seems most likely to succeed.

Both inpatient and outpatient facilities have their pros and cons. Outpatient programs tend to be much less expensive and time-demanding for patients. Patients learn lifestyle changes to help them cope better with pain, while also staying in touch with normal life at home and work. On the other hand, an inpatient program can work with patients more intensely to help them learn ways to alter negative behavior and attitudes related to their pain. What's more, if part of their pain stems from tensions at home, an inpatient program could offer breathing space—a chance to rethink what goes on at home and to learn new ways of handling it.

STUDIES ON EFFECTIVENESS OF PAIN CLINICS

How effective are pain clinics in helping people with chronic pain? Most of the research studies attempting to answer that question have focused on multidisciplinary pain clinics and centers.

When pain clinics began to appear in the United States, many health professionals doubted these facilities could make any real difference. The assumption was that the multidisciplinary team approach was expensive and no more successful than

History of Pain Clinics

Most pain experts trace the origin of pain clinics to post-World War II England, where facilities were set up to help soldiers deal with severe pain resulting from war injuries. Other pain clinics emerged in the 1950s, usually based on the application of the techniques of anesthesiology to pain relief. Also in the 1950s, John Bonica, M.D., who is considered the father of modern pain management, pioneered a different strategy. Rather than viewing pain patients as people who needed something "fixed" by a doctor, these new clinics focused on the idea that the patients themselves needed to take responsibility for their treatment and its outcome. They were treated with the goal of returning to a more normal lifestyle, not of "curing" their pain.

other pain treatment programs. But studies refuting those doubts soon began to emerge.

For instance, a research team at the New Hope Pain Center in California followed 151 former patients to determine if treatment had long-term success. The researchers reported in 1981 in the *National Institute on Drug Abuse Research Monograph* that:

• After four years, 38 percent of the patients were using no barbiturates, muscle relaxants, opioids, or tranquilizers. Thirty-one percent were using less medication than before treatment.

- After four years, 85 percent had had no invasive or medical treatment for their pain.
- At the one-year and four-year points, about 50 percent said their pain was better than it was before admission to the clinic.
- 75 percent of the patients reported positive attitudes, both in regard to their pain and their general lifestyle.

Other studies of the effectiveness of pain clinics have zeroed in on just one factor: whether people were able to return to work. A research team at the Comprehensive Pain and Rehabilitation Center, affiliated with the University of Miami School of Medicine in Florida, did a review and meta-analysis of 37 research studies of this type. (A meta-analysis uses statistical methods to combine results of different studies.) Reporting in a 1994 issue of *Spine*, the Florida researchers found that:

- Nonsurgical treatment of chronic pain did help patients return to work; an average of 38 percent were working at the time of follow-up (pain had prevented all of them from working before treatment).
- Benefits of the pain-clinic treatment programs were not just temporary, but still evident at follow-up, which averaged 14 months after treatment.
- Increased rates of return to work were due to treatment at the pain clinics.

Healing the Pain

FINDING A PAIN CLINIC

If you think a pain clinic might be a good option for you, talk it over with your doctor, who should be able to steer you to a reputable, professionally staffed pain clinic in your area. You may want to do a little additional checking on your own to be absolutely comfortable with the facility's credentials.

Your physician should also be kept informed of your progress once you've enrolled. When you finish the program, your doctor should play a role in your follow-up care and in supporting and encouraging you to continue with your newly learned pain-management skills.

Considering the abundance of programs that have surfaced in recent years, all under the umbrella of "pain clinic," be sure to carefully evaluate the quality of the facility. Seek a second opinion if you encounter a clinic representative who is eager to perform surgery, prescribes lots of medications, or makes inflated promises about curing your pain.

Healing the Pain

CHAPTER 12
Physical and
Occupational Therapy

Physical and occupational therapy both help people regain or improve physical functioning. There are some differences, however, in how physical and occupational therapists are trained and in the focus of their practice.

Physical therapy involves "the assessment, evaluation, treatment, and prevention of physical disability, movement dysfunctions, and pain resulting from injury, disease, disability, or other health-related conditions," according to the textbook *Introduction to Physical Therapy.* Occupational therapy, on the other hand, concentrates more on "therapeutic use of self-care, work, and play activities to increase independent function, enhance development, and prevent disability. [It] may include adaptation of task or environment to achieve maximum independence and to enhance quality of life," according to the Representative Assembly of the American Occupational Therapy Association.

In reality, however, the lines can't be drawn so distinctly between the two professions. Physical therapists may teach people daily living activities, such as eating or dressing, just as occupational therapists do. And the occupational therapist working on an activity with a patient suffering from a painful condition often uses such treatment methods as massage and heat, just as physical therapists do.

The differences between the two professions, then, are not so important. In treating painful conditions, physical and occupational therapy clearly play complementary roles. Therapists from both disciplines are often represented on the teams of many pain clinics that take a multidisciplinary approach to pain treatment (see the chapter on Pain Clinics).

PHYSICAL THERAPY AND PAIN

Pain is a major reason that people seek physical therapy. Both acute pain (such as injury-induced pain or postsurgical pain) and chronic pain (which may begin as acute pain or develop gradually, lasting longer than expected for normal healing) are targeted by physical therapists. In the case of acute pain, the therapist aims to prevent more serious injury or impairment and quickly return the patient to normal daily life. For chronic pain, the goal is to restore functioning through a more prolonged, progressive approach.

In general, the physical therapist focuses on evaluating and treating the underlying physical abnormality responsible for the pain. Sometimes, however, the underlying problem can't be completely corrected. In that case, the physical therapist's goal is to reduce the pain and disability and restore as much normal functioning as possible.

Healing the Pain

At one time, physical therapy consisted mostly of passive techniques. But research has found that more active methods are crucial to prevent physical deterioration, return lost functioning, and build strength in pain patients. Physical therapists now use both passive and active treatment techniques. Passive methods include massage, heat therapy, and gentle movement of painful joints to increase range of motion.

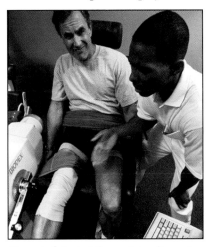
The goal of physical therapy is to relieve pain, build strength, and restore normal functioning.

Below is a list of treatments a physical therapist might use to treat patients experiencing pain. You'll find more information on several of these treatment options in other chapters of this book.

- Assistive or adaptive equipment: explaining and demonstrating how to use devices such as a cane, a supportive neck collar, crutches, lumbar supports, a walker, and a wheelchair
- Biofeedback: teaching techniques to control body functions—such as heart rate, breathing, and muscle tension—and thus also to manage pain
- Cryotherapy: using cold temperatures in a therapeutic way, such as application of ice packs

- Electric current: applying electric current, as with transcutaneous electrical nerve stimulation (TENS)
- Electromagnetic radiation: inducing therapeutic deep heat through the use of electromagnetic energy to elevate the body's temperature
- Exercise: teaching appropriate movements to enhance the range of motion, increase strength, and reduce pain
- Hydrotherapy: using water for therapy, as in a whirlpool or a simple hot bath

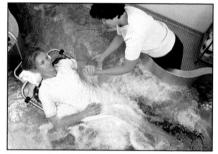

Whirlpool baths help relax stiff or injured muscles, easing pain and making physical therapy easier to perform.

- Massage: relaxing muscles through stretching, rubbing, and other manipulation techniques
- Mechanical compression: applying pressure to decrease swelling
- Mobilization: restoring normal movement through manual techniques
- Orthoses: supporting joints through the use of braces, splints, foot supports, and similar devices
- Posture training: providing instruction in proper body alignment for common activities such as sitting at a desk, relaxing on the sofa, ironing, and washing dishes

Healing the Pain

- Traction: pulling, or distraction, of joints through manual or mechanical means, or a combination of the two

Any physical therapy program must include patient education in pain-control techniques and body mechanics, as well as a home exercise program to help maintain the gains made in therapy. Patients themselves learn how to help their condition and what they can do to avoid aggravating their pain.

Physical therapy also can sometimes help patients avoid the discomfort and cost of surgery. A Norwegian study published in the *British Medical Journal* in 1993, for example, reported that physical therapy alone was just as helpful as arthroscopic surgery to patients with rotator cuff disease, a painful condition resulting from inflammation of the tendons around the shoulder joint.

And a study of back-pain patients found that those who completed a physical therapy program fared much better than those who hadn't. At a two-year follow-up point, 87 percent of the patients who had received physical therapy had returned to work as compared with only 41 percent who had not received physical therapy, according to a report in a 1987 issue of the *Journal of the American Medical Association*. Moreover, twice as many patients who hadn't had physical therapy had undergone spinal operations.

More research is needed on the role of physical therapy in pain rehabilitation and prevention. Upcoming studies funded

Healing the Pain

by the Foundation for Physical Therapy, focusing on such conditions as back injury and carpal tunnel syndrome, should shed more light on this issue.

OCCUPATIONAL THERAPY AND PAIN

Occupational therapists treat people with acute and chronic pain conditions that get in the way of performing work-related and other daily activities. This kind of therapy is based on the premise that occupation—whether that of a child playing or going to school, an adult working

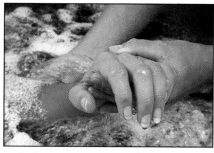

Hydrotherapy is especially beneficial to those suffering from joint ailments. The water gently massages the injured limb and also helps support it.

at a job or enjoying a round of golf, or an elderly person retaining the ability to live independently—has a profound effect on a person's health. Occupational therapists primarily work on activities that restore or enhance the ability to work, do normal day-to-day tasks around the home or out in the community, and enjoy leisure pastimes. While working with pain patients, occupational therapists may use pain treatments (such as cold, heat, and hydrotherapy) to minimize the patient's discomfort in doing the activities.

Occupational therapy professionals use four primary methods in their work:

Therapeutic use of self. The therapist's caring, understanding, and acceptance of the patient form the basis of the therapeutic relationship.

Purposeful activity. Through purposeful activity, human beings influence their own physical, mental, and emotional health and have an impact on their social and physical surroundings. Activity both prevents and treats dysfunctions. Occupational therapists use a wide range of activities with their patients to help develop physical, cognitive, psychological, and social functioning. Pottery making, basketry, industrial tooling, photography, and computer skills are just a few examples of such activities. Self-care skills, such as dressing and personal hygiene, are also taught. Clearly, these purposeful activities are diverse, but some characteristics are common to all of them:

- They are goal-directed.
- They are meaningful. The activity has to have some value to the individual, even if it is not realized immediately.
- They get the client actively involved.
- They are geared to improving function and preventing malfunction.
- They relate to life tasks. Self-care, work, or leisure activities all aim to build skills essential in the various life roles of the client.
- They tie into a client's interests.

Healing the Pain

Activity analysis. This consists of evaluating an activity to determine its therapeutic potential. It addresses questions such as "What movements, skills, or abilities are crucial to performing an activity?" and "Is the client ready to tackle them?"

Activity adaptation. Some changes may be required in the activity itself, or to the environment in which it's performed, in order to accommodate an individual patient. It's especially crucial to stretch the client with a manageable challenge without pushing too hard, which might cause frustration and, as a result, bring therapy to an end.

FINDING A PHYSICAL THERAPIST OR OCCUPATIONAL THERAPIST

Both physical therapists and occupational therapists must earn four-year college degrees from accredited programs. Masters and doctorate degrees also are available. Most states require both types of therapists to obtain a license to practice.

If you would like to engage the services of a physical or occupational therapist, ask your health care provider for a suggestion. In 30 states, physician referrals are not necessary to secure treatment. Today, many physical and occupational therapists work out of private practice, as well as in hospitals and pain clinics. As with other licensed health care professionals, local and state associations can provide you with a list of therapists in your area.

CHAPTER 13
Prescription Medications

In the battle against pain, prescription medications are a potent weapon. As scientists continue to study pain, their increased understanding will allow them to concoct new medications to help thwart its physiologic discomfort. In the future we can expect more effective and safer pain remedies—both in terms of the medications themselves and in the ways they are administered.

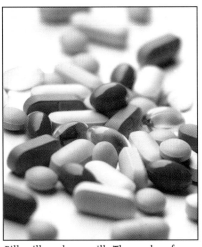

We're lucky to live at a time when we have more medicinal answers to pain, yet as consumers we need to be better informed and more assertive than ever before. Indeed, that's where

Pills, pills, and more pills. The number of prescription medications for physicians to choose from keeps growing every year.

it gets complicated. The array of prescription medications keeps expanding. Their health benefits are touted, but we also hear about their risks and side effects as well as the negative interactions between medicines (both prescription and non-prescription), and between prescription medications and tobacco, alcohol, dietary supplements, and even food. The scenario is ripe for confusion. Consider these statistics:

- As of the mid-1990s, pharmacists in the United States were dispensing more than 2 billion prescriptions a year.
- Experts estimate that from 30 to 50 percent of patients fail to use their prescription medicines properly.
- Misuse of medications and adverse reactions to them cost an estimated $20 billion a year in medical bills. Add the resulting expense due to lost productivity, and the cost jumps to $100 billion annually.

Clearly, it's in your best interests to know as much as you can about the prescriptions you are taking, whether for pain or some other health condition. To reduce possible risks, become informed about what those prescriptions are, what benefits you can expect from them, and how to use them properly.

TYPES OF PRESCRIPTION PAIN MEDICATIONS

Dozens of prescription pain medications are now on the market, with many more in some state of research, development, or testing. Discussing them all would fill a book by itself. Our review is limited to the main categories of prescription pain remedies.

NSAIDs. Nonsteroidal anti-inflammatory drugs (NSAIDs) relieve pain by inhibiting the production of prostaglandins, which are chemicals in the body that cause inflammation and trigger the transmission of pain signals to the brain. NSAIDs are used to help relieve many types of pain, ranging from the common headache to mild cancer pain. Because of their anti-inflammatory properties, NSAIDs are especially effective in treating pain and inflammation from conditions such as arthritis and muscle sprains.

NSAIDs are often preferred to corticosteroids (pain relievers that contain cortisone) because long-term use of corticosteroids can lead to potentially serious adverse effects (see "Corticosteroids," p. 123). NSAIDs don't pose those risks, but they do have a few undesirable side effects of their own. For example, researchers have linked NSAIDs to gastrointestinal bleeding and kidney damage. Lower-dosage forms of NSAIDs are readily available without a prescription. (See the chapter on over-the-counter medications for more on NSAIDs.)

Narcotics. These medications work for moderate to severe pain, such as that which accompanies cancer or which follows surgery. Some possible side effects from narcotics include constipation, depression of breathing, drowsiness, mood changes, nausea, difficulty urinating, and vomiting.

Many patients and some doctors are afraid that narcotics are addictive and therefore avoid the medication. But other pain experts believe these fears are exaggerated and prevent some patients with severe pain from getting maximum relief. The differing opinions come from a widespread confusion about the difference between *physical dependence* and *addiction*. Long-term use of narcotics can lead to tolerance—that is, over time patients may require higher doses to achieve the same amount of pain relief. But this rarely leads to addiction in people who have not had a tendency toward addiction before treatment. *Physical dependence* means the patient will experience withdrawal symptoms if the narcotic-based medication is stopped abruptly, although a gradual reduction generally eliminates the problem. Physical dependence is quite different from *addiction*, which is characterized by an unrelenting craving for and obsession with getting more drugs. And that involves an individual's personality and life circumstances. After all, drugs are used by addicts for psychological reasons, for getting "high," not for pain relief. Although few patients who take narcotics for pain relief develop an addiction, considerations of tolerance, physical dependence, and addiction are genuine issues and a source of controversy among pain-relief specialists.

Antidepressants. As the name implies, these medications are primarily used to treat depression. However, some antidepressants may also provide relief to those suffering from chronic pain, even if they aren't depressed. Some antidepressants have proved useful in the treatment of neuropathic (nerve injury), head, and cancer pain. Side effects of these medications may include constipation, dizziness when standing up suddenly, drowsiness, and dry mouth.

Anticonvulsants. These drugs were originally developed to control seizures and other symptoms of epilepsy, but they also are effective for treating chronic nerve pain in some patients. Adverse effects can include disorientation and drowsiness and possibly interference with liver and blood-cell function.

Corticosteroids. Known to most people simply as "steroids," these medications reduce pain caused by swelling and inflammation. For cancer patients, steroids also relieve bone pain and pain caused by brain and spinal-cord tumors. Side effects can include bleeding, confusion, fluid buildup, and stomach irritation. Prolonged use can lead to many problems, including cataracts, diabetes mellitus, high blood pressure, immune system impairment, osteoporosis, and severe mental or behavioral disturbances.

Other medications. Other commonly used prescription pain relievers don't readily fit into any of the above categories. For example: Sumatriptan is often prescribed for migraine headaches (though it must be avoided by people with heart disease or uncontrolled high blood pressure). Capsaicin is made from red-pepper extract; when applied to the skin it can alleviate pain from cluster headache, various types of neuralgias (nerve-pain disorders), osteoarthritis, post-mastectomy pain, rheumatoid arthritis, and shingles.

NOT JUST PILLS AND SHOTS

Pain medications can now be effectively delivered to the body by a number of innovative methods:

Lollipops. These are especially effective for children, but adults also use them for pain control. Lollipops are available with fentanyl, which is a narcotic. Absorbed through the mucous membranes of the mouth, fentanyl serves as a premedication (administered prior to medical procedures likely to cause pain), for the relief of pain after surgery or serious injury, and for severe cancer-related pain. The pain lollipop is only available for use in hospital settings.

Transdermal patch. Applied to the surface of the skin, a transdermal patch delivers medication to the bloodstream by absorption through the skin. Fentanyl (sold under the brand name Duragesic) is one example of a drug available in patch form; it is suitable for people who are unable to take medication by mouth and is especially useful

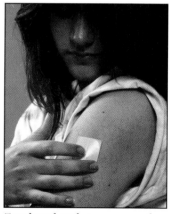

Transdermal patches are worn on the skin, which absorbs the medication.

Healing the Pain

Other Innovations on the Way

Medical research continues its search for more effective pain medications and better ways to deliver them. Here are a few new ideas under development:

- Scientists are working on a button-size implanted device, placed just under the skin, that can deliver painkiller into the bloodstream continuously for three months. Tests with cancer patients should be underway by the time you read this.

- New drugs, such as DuP 747, may work to relieve pain as well as morphine and other narcotics do, but without the sedation and other side effects.

- Yet another approach is to develop pain relievers that boost production of the body's own natural painkilling chemicals, such as endorphins and enkephalins. Again, widespread testing will be required.

for those experiencing constant pain, such as pain caused by cancer, rather than for quick pain relief.

Bedside pump. Used mostly in hospitals, the pump uses an intravenous tube to allow a patient to push a button to receive a pre-set dose of medication that has been programmed by a physician or nurse. The pump lets the patient feel more in control of his or her own pain relief. It also avoids delays in receiving medication that arise in busy hospitals. This type of device is commonly used for patients with pain due to cancer, surgery, or trauma.

Smaller portable pumps. Computerized pump devices the size of a handheld tape recorder can be worn on a person's belt, so they go with the patient anywhere. Pushing a button delivers a pre-set dose of pain medication intravenously. Again, dosage and interval are programmed and locked into the device by a physician or nurse. Such pumps can spare severe chronic-pain sufferers repeated trips to hospital emergency rooms for injections of pain relievers.

Implantable pumps. Smaller still are the newer implantable pumps. These are about the size of a yo-yo and are surgically implanted under the skin. From there, they deliver painkilling medication very close to the pain-control centers in the spinal cord or brain, thus requiring lower dosages than oral administration. For some select patients with severe pain, implantable pumps have provided better relief without the serious side effects of some oral medications. But implantable pumps are quite expensive (costing as much as $25,000), must be replaced every three to five years, and have their own risks and complications.

Despite all these innovative techniques, some forms of pain simply cannot be relieved: Even high-dose narcotics and pumps may not be effective against pain caused by nerve damage.

Healing the Pain

SMART USAGE DEPENDS ON YOU

Pain medication has risks as well as benefits. To minimize the former and get the most of the latter, you need to ask many questions. Here is a starter list developed by the National Council on Patient Information and Education in Washington, D.C.:

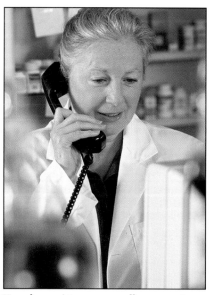

Your pharmacist can answer all your questions about prescription medications and ensure that you use them properly and effectively.

- What is this medicine's correct name, and what is it supposed to do?
- How much time is required for the drug to take effect?
- How and when do I take it, and for how long?
- Do you have written information about this medicine?
- What foods, drinks, activities, or other medicines should I avoid while taking this medicine?
- What are the side effects, and how do I respond to them?
- Will this new prescription work safely with the other prescription and over-the-counter medications I'm taking? (Take along all the containers of medication you're currently using so the doctor will be able to answer this question.)

Write down the answers to each question to help you remember all the details after you leave the physician's office or the pharmacy. If there's something you didn't understand the first time through, don't be afraid to ask for clarification. If you're hard of hearing, ask for legibly written instructions or bring a companion along who can write them down for you.

Remember, asking questions does not mean you're being a nuisance. An all-too-common perception among patients is that health care providers are always in a hurry, and you shouldn't slow them down with your questions. On the contrary, keep in mind that you are paying for the provider's services. You have a right to ask questions and the provider has a duty to answer them. In fact, for your own health and safety, you have an obligation to ask questions. If your health care provider never seems willing to spend enough time to answer your questions, perhaps it's time to look for a new provider.

If you take a number of prescriptions, it's a good idea to always use the same pharmacy. Getting to know the pharmacists will make you feel more comfortable about asking questions. They'll also get to know you and learn how best to be of service to you.

If you'd like more information, visit a bookstore or library for a reference book on prescription drugs. Look for one that gives a complete description of your medications, including what they're supposed to do, side effects, adverse reactions and interactions, recommended dosages, and warnings.

Healing the Pain

CHAPTER 14
Support Groups

The English poet and essayist Samuel Johnson (1709–1784) once said, "Those who do not feel pain seldom think that it is felt." If you're living with chronic pain, you know exactly what Johnson meant. As understanding as family, friends, and co-workers may try to be, they can't fully comprehend what you're going through unless they've had a comparable experience.

Support groups, also known as peer-support or self-help groups, first became popular in the 1970s as a way to provide the emotional support and empathy that friends and relatives cannot. Through these groups, millions of people have gained the courage and confidence to confront serious life problems, from divorce to drug addiction to a fatal illness. People living with chronic pain have also turned to support groups. By the early 1980s, an estimated half-million support groups existed in the United States alone.

DO SUPPORT GROUPS REALLY HELP?

Support groups first gained credibility in the treatment of serious illness in 1989. That year Dr. David Spiegel of the Stanford University School of Medicine published a landmark study showing that women with advanced breast cancer had benefited from weekly support-group sessions that also included instruction in self-hypnosis for pain control. At the end of one year, the women reported less anxiety, less depression, and less pain than women in a control group that only received medical treatment.

What surprised Spiegel the most, however, came four years later when he did a follow-up study. He found that women who were part of the support group had survived twice as long as those in the control group—about 18 months longer, on average. In fact, one-third of the members of the support group were still alive four years after the study began. Everyone in the medical-treatment-only group had died.

The medical world took notice, and other studies have since replicated Spiegel's findings. In fact, in a commentary in a 1995 issue of *Public Health Reports*, Spiegel points out that the question is no longer whether psychological approaches work in helping people with health problems, but rather which ones work best.

How Support Relates to Health

No one knows exactly how support groups affect health. But we do know that people with chronic pain or other physical problems often become isolated from others. Support groups help counteract that isolation, providing a place for you to talk with people who are going through similar experiences— people who hardly need an explanation about what you're going through. Just knowing that you're not alone, that other people have the same frustrations, stresses, and concerns as you do, can be an enormous source of comfort and relief.

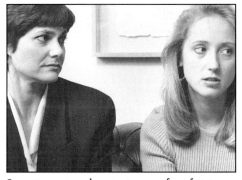

Support groups can be a great source of comfort to those suffering from chronic pain. And the emotional support often translates into improved health.

In addition to feeling less isolated, people in support groups develop a connection to others that is likely to bolster their confidence and increase their motivation and their ability to cope. Helping others in the group also adds to feelings of self-worth. Group members learn tips about coping skills from each other, which is a crucial aspect for people with chronic pain. The group is not just a place to talk about how much it hurts, but an opportunity to learn how to handle pain better.

The "grandmother effect" is another theory developed to explain the benefit of support groups. This theory claims that when people feel others care about them, they are more likely to care about themselves. That may translate into better health practices, such as getting exercise, eating well, sleeping well, and avoiding self-destructive habits. In turn, those practices may boost a person's ability to fight illness, dysfunction, or pain. And the social connection in the group may make it easier to communicate effectively with health care providers.

A sense of connection to others also might actually serve to protect you against the physiologic effects of stress on the body. Stress hormones may worsen physical illness and pain. In turn, illness and pain trigger the production of more stress hormones, leading to even more pain and illness. Any activity that keeps stress hormones in check would help to break this spiraling effect.

Some of the difficulty in assessing the effectiveness of support groups is that they are often part of a more comprehensive program to help people cope with pain or illness. In addition to participating in a support group, participants might engage in relaxation techniques, hypnosis, exercise, dietary changes, or other therapies. Studies have shown that all these approaches can be effective in coping with pain and improving health. Thus, it's hard to pinpoint the benefits of support groups alone.

Could it be that these elements together have more benefit than any single element does by itself—that, in effect, the whole is greater than the sum of the parts? Perhaps. At any rate, we still have much to learn about how social support plays a role in a person's health.

MANY FORMS OF SUPPORT GROUPS

Support groups take many forms. Some meet face to face, others interact via telephone lines, computer bulletin boards, or networks. Some are organized by psychologists, doctors, and other health care providers, whereas sometimes participants

The Price of Isolation

One fundamental benefit of support groups is combating the social isolation people in chronic pain may feel. Indeed, social isolation may have consequences beyond just feeling lonely, according to findings of several scientific studies. For instance, in 1988, University of Michigan researchers reported in *Science* that social isolation posed as serious a risk for illness and early death as smoking, high blood pressure, high cholesterol, obesity, and sedentary lifestyle. Other studies in the United States and Europe have come to similar conclusions.

launch the group. Some groups are structured; others are more informal. Groups may take an educational approach or be largely social. They may meet in clinic or hospital settings, in community facilities such as libraries, or even in someone's living room.

Support groups sometimes take on a role beyond what is typically viewed as "support." For instance, they may present public seminars to raise awareness about a specific health problem, invite expert speakers to talk to members and families, send out newsletters to share information, or set up a speakers' bureau for community outreach.

Whatever form they take, support groups can be a real bargain. Most are free of charge, although some may have a nom-

Healing the Pain

inal fee to cover incidental costs, such as newsletter production, mailings, and space rental.

Choosing a Support Group

First of all, remember that support groups are a complement to professional health care, not a replacement for it. Be clear with yourself about what you can expect to get out of this kind of group.

Keep in mind that support groups aren't the answer for everyone. If you're extremely shy, the experience may cause anxiety. And if you easily become distraught listening to other people's problems, a support group could be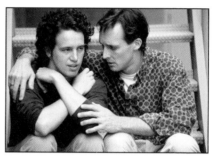

You are the best judge of whether a support group will be of benefit. For some, a close, attentive friend is a better solution.

too stressful. Some people prefer the comfort of a single close friend or even solitude when sorting out their problems.

If you feel that a support group for chronic pain might be a positive experience for you, here are some points to consider:

• Does the group include people who have lived with the pain problem for a long time as well as those just beginning to cope? Veterans of pain can speak from the wisdom of experience, while newcomers bring in fresh perspectives.

- If the group has a leader, is it someone who positively influences the group discussion? Do shy people receive encouragement? Are the more outgoing or domineering people restrained from taking over the group?
- In general, is this a group of people you think you feel comfortable with?
- Does it seem this group will be around for a while, and does it meet frequently enough to satisfy your needs?
- Are members who have been in the group for a while truly benefiting from their participation? After your first or second session, talk with others one-on-one to find out what they have gained from their experience with the group.

Be alert to these *warning signals* before getting involved in a particular group:

- Promises of quick fixes or miracle cures
- Sales pitches to encourage you to buy particular products
- Too much focus on airing complaints, not enough on constructive discussion
- Suggestions that you stop other forms of treatment to concentrate exclusively on the group
- Too many prying questions that make you feel uncomfortable (but you should expect to hear some unsettling questions and comments now and then, since you'll be talking about sensitive issues)
- High membership fees

Healing the Pain

- Advocating one method as "the answer" to your pain problem
- Any trappings of cultism

FINDING A SUPPORT GROUP

A good place to start is with your own health care provider, who may know of support groups designed for people with your kind of pain. You can also contact local clinics, hospitals, and wellness programs to find out about groups they offer.

For other leads, watch community bulletin boards, local newspapers, other media sources, and the World Wide Web. Associations for specific health problems—such as the American Cancer Society or the National Headache Foundation—may be able to steer you to local support groups, too. Check your phone book for state or local chapters or ask your librarian for help. Finally, if you are unable to find a support group in your area, consider organizing one yourself.

If you need additional help in locating or organizing a support group, contact the organization listed below:

> **American Self-Help Clearinghouse**
> **Northwest Covenant Medical Center**
>
> 25 Pocono Road
> Denville, NJ 07834
> 201-625-7101

CHAPTER 15
Surgery

Surgery is a complicated, highly technical, invasive, and expensive procedure, as well as a distressing one. When it comes to treating pain, surgery usually is the last resort. If your doctor recommends surgery, ask lots of questions about the proposed operation, such as:

- What is surgery expected to do for me?
- Why is surgery recommended over other treatment options?
- What are the risks of the surgery?
- What degree of pain relief can I expect from the operation?
- Will I be prevented from carrying on my normal daily activities? If so, how will I be limited and for how long?
- What success rates for this surgery have been reported in

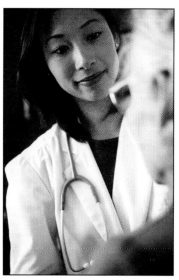

A good doctor will take the time to listen to and answer all your questions about a proposed operation.

the medical literature? (Don't rely on the doctor's personal anecdotal reports of success; ask for specific research findings.) And exactly what is meant by "success"? Does it refer to less pain at one month? Six months? Five years?

- How long is the recovery period?
- If I go ahead with this surgery, what are the chances that I will need one or more additional operations later on?

Your health care provider should be straightforward in answering your questions. You should also get a second opinion to help determine if surgery is the wisest choice for you. If you decide to have the operation, be sure to check out the surgeon's credentials. Find out how often he or she has performed this particular procedure before, and how recently.

TYPES OF SURGERY FOR PAIN RELIEF

Just as there are many types of pain, so there are numerous surgical procedures for relieving pain. In general, surgery aims to provide pain relief through one of the following approaches:

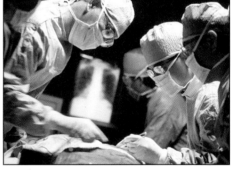

Although no one's favorite alternative, surgery sometimes is the only way to treat the underlying cause of your pain.

Anatomic. An anatomic procedure deals directly with the structural problem causing the pain. If compression on a nerve is the source of pain, for example, the purpose of surgery would be to reduce or eliminate the cause of the compression.

Modulatory. These surgical procedures use electrical stimulation or chemicals to interfere with the transmission of pain signals to the brain. For instance, a programmable device that sends electrical impulses to electrodes next to the spinal cord can be surgically implanted (in a procedure similar to implanting a pacemaker for the heart). Or, a pump can be implanted inside the body to send pain-relieving medications directly into the fluid around the spinal cord.

Destructive (or ablative). These are procedures that destroy portions of the nervous system to block the transmission of pain signals. Because destructive procedures are irreversible, they are used only for severe pain in serious circumstances when no other course of action is likely to alleviate the problem. They are usually reserved for patients with a short life expectancy.

SURGERY FOR A FEW PAINFUL CONDITIONS

Dozens of pain-surgery techniques are in use today; we can't begin to cover them all here. Many of these procedures are used primarily for severe conditions, such as to relieve the pain of cancer patients who have a limited life expectancy.

In the rest of this chapter we will consider the usefulness of surgery for three less serious, but fairly common, painful con-

ditions: back pain, carpal tunnel syndrome, and temporomandibular disorders. Our discussion will summarize current
thinking on these procedures, but bear in mind that surgery
always has been and remains an evolving technology, with surgeons continually modifying old procedures and developing
new ones to achieve the best results.

BACK PAIN

Odds are that at some point in your life you will have back
pain severe enough to require medical help. Back pain is the
second most frequent reason people see a doctor (the common cold is first). It is the third most common reason that
people end up on the operating table.

Back surgery may be common, but it's highly controversial
in the medical community. This controversy was epitomized
by the furor over the practice guidelines on low-back problems in adults, which were released by the Agency for Health
Care Policy Research (AHCPR) in 1994. The purpose of the
AHCPR is to survey the medical literature to determine the
effectiveness of common medical procedures. According to the
AHCPR's report, surgery was unnecessary in almost all cases
when back pain lasted less than three months.

A group of back surgeons from across the nation blasted
AHCPR for its findings and immediately formed a lobbying
group to urge Congress to drastically cut the agency's budget.
Their efforts were unsuccessful, for the most part. But the

Healing the Pain

furor that broke out illustrates how divided the medical profession is over the question of back surgery.

That leaves the health care consumer in a quandary. Which advice do you believe?

There are no easy answers. But for starters, bear in mind that the vast majority of people with back pain will never need surgery. In most cases, back pain eventually vanishes. And usually only low-tech treatments—such as exercise or over-the-counter medications—are needed.

Back surgery is clearly necessary, however, when back pain is accompanied by the sudden onset of leg problems and loss of bowel and bladder control. These are symptoms of *cauda equina* compression, which requires immediate surgery to prevent permanent nerve damage.

Sciatica, which manifests itself as a shooting pain down the leg, is a condition that may or may not call for surgery. The chief cause of sciatica is a herniated disk (commonly called a slipped disk) of the lower back. A herniation occurs when the outer fibrous ring breaks down and the gelatinlike center of the disk bulges out through the disk's outer covering. The fibrous ring or the center material may compress a spinal nerve, causing pain. But a bout with sciatica doesn't automatically mean a herniated disk or surgery. Almost all doctors advocate waiting at least a month.

Medical research showing that many people with disk abnormalities do not experience back pain supports the wait-

and-see approach. A 1994 study in the *New England Journal of Medicine* looked at the MRI (magnetic resonance imaging) scans of 98 people with no back pain. Only 36 percent had completely normal disks, with the MRIs of the others showing disk bulges or protrusions. In fact, researchers have found that even young adults have bulging disks, but no signs of back pain. Such findings raise the question: Is there a cause-and-effect connection between disk abnormalities and back pain, or is it merely a matter of coincidence?

The upshot of all this is that the appearance of an abnormal disk on an MRI or other diagnostic image is not reason enough to justify back surgery.

Sometimes, however, back pain doesn't subside after four to six weeks. Surgery may be appropriate in some of these cases. The following are among the possible surgical procedures for relieving nerve compression:

Aspiration percutaneous lumbar diskectomy. In this procedure, the surgeon inserts a large needle through the patient's skin. A device inside the needle is then used to loosen or remove the damaged disk.

Laminectomy and diskectomy. The surgeon removes pieces of the disk that are pressing on the sciatic nerve root.

An alternative to surgery is a process called chemonucleolysis, in which the doctor injects chymopapain (an enzyme from the papaya fruit) into the affected disk. The enzyme eats away at the disk bulge, taking the pressure off the squeezed nerve. But here again, medical experts disagree on the effectiveness of this procedure. Some surgeons are reluctant to use it because of risks of nerve damage and allergic reactions to the enzyme. Others, including a group of British researchers reporting in a 1996 issue of *Spine*, claim it's effective. They found chymopapain to work just as well as surgery in treating 42 teenagers with back pain due to disk protrusions. These researchers suggested reserving surgery for those who get no help from the chymopapain.

Carpal tunnel syndrome

This is a type of overuse strain injury or repetitive-motion syndrome. The carpal tunnel is a passageway formed by the wrist bones and the band of connective tissue known as the transverse carpal ligament. Inside this tunnel are the median nerve and the tendons that allow you to bend your fingers and thumb. Repeated grasping, pinching, gripping, twisting, and turning movements of the hands and wrists can cause the lining of the carpal tunnel membrane to swell, squeezing the median nerve and causing numbness, tingling, or pain in the palm, thumb, first three fingers, or back toward the elbow.

A surgical correction of this problem, called carpal tunnel decompression, involves dividing the carpal ligament to relieve pressure on the median nerve. Again, most medical

Healing the Pain

experts recommend surgery only when other pain-relief treatments have been unsuccessful.

When surgery is necessary, some doctors report good results with endoscopic procedures, in which an instrument is used to visualize the interior of a body part. A study in the *Canadian Journal of Surgery* in 1994 reported on 95 patients who had endured symptoms for an average of nearly four years. All had previously undergone nonsurgical treatments, including splinting, nonsteroidal anti-inflammatory drugs (NSAIDs), and steroid injections, without adequate relief. After surgery, all but 6 of the 95 reported pain relief. Of the 61 patients in the group who had jobs, 52 returned to work without restriction. Four patients developed complications from the surgery.

This doesn't mean endoscopic surgery is the only surgical option. The most common operation is a ten-minute procedure involving open surgery and is effective for many patients. For more on carpal tunnel syndrome, see pages 168–171.

TEMPOROMANDIBULAR DISORDERS

Jaw pain, facial and neck-muscle pain, headaches, toothaches, and earaches can all be part of the discomfort of temporomandibular disorders, or TMD. Although TMD has received a lot of attention in recent years, from both the medical community and the general public, it remains a disorder surrounded by uncertainty. Such was the conclusion of a mid-1996 scientific conference on TMD convened by the National

Institutes of Health(NIH). A panel of experts surveyed the scientific evidence to date and reported that "scientifically based guidelines for diagnosis and management of TMD are still unavailable." In particular, questions were raised about certain types of aggressive treatments for TMD.

One surgical procedure that led to disastrous results was the Vitek jaw implant. This is a Teflon-laminated device that had been inserted into the jaw joint as a shock absorber intended to replace the cartilage disk that normally serves this function. Not long after this implant was first introduced, however, reports of trouble began to surface. The normal pressures of chewing caused the implant to break into small pieces, triggering a biochemical reaction that damaged the jawbone. Although the Vitek implant was removed from the market in 1988, by that time thousands of people who had already received implants were permanently disfigured and disabled.

After such experiences, doctors and patients alike have been skeptical of other TMD surgery. Today, medical experts remain sharply divided in their opinions of surgery's usefulness. But they do seem to agree on one point, according to the NIH conference panel: Surgery should be considered for TMD only when all other options have been exhausted. The panel advised trying conservative treatments first, such as physical therapy, stress reduction, the use of pain-relieving medications, and the sharp reduction or outright elimination of gum chewing.

For more on TMD, see pages 235–239.

CHAPTER 16

Transcutaneous Electrical Nerve Stimulation (TENS)

Transcutaneous electrical nerve stimulation, or TENS, is based on the theory that stimulating nerve fibers can relieve pain by blocking, or "closing the gate on," signals to the brain. It is a fairly simple technology that uses a battery-powered transmitter the size of a small transistor radio, plus electrodes and cable wires, to send low-intensity electrical impulses through the skin to the targeted nerves beneath. Pain relief usually begins within a few minutes, and the patient can regulate the controls as needed during treatment.

TENS units are pocket-sized, making them easy to carry around. Pain relief, then, is available wherever and whenever you need it.

Because the transmitter is so small, a patient can wear the TENS unit on a belt or clipped onto a pocket, making it possible to receive treatment while going about normal daily activities. Therapy sessions usually last at least a couple of hours, sometimes longer, depending on the nature of the pain. TENS also offers the advantages of being noninvasive, generally safe (but see some cautions below), and controlled by the patient. Using TENS may also reduce the need for pain medications.

No one knows for sure how or why TENS works. Besides the "gate control" theory mentioned earlier, it's possible that, like acupuncture, TENS may increase the body's production of endorphins, natural pain-relieving substances. Sometimes practitioners place TENS electrodes over acupuncture meridian points (for more on meridians, see the chapter on acupuncture) to increase the effectiveness of the treatment. This is sometimes referred to as *Acupuncture-TENS*.

Today, physicians, nurses, physical therapists, chiropractors, naturopathic doctors, and other health practitioners use TENS as a pain-relief tool. Because it is portable and easy to use, patients can use this therapy in the hospital, clinic, or home. TENS is used for pain such as:

- Arthritis
- Cancer pain
- Dental pain
- Dysmenorrhea (painful menstruation)
- Fibromyalgia (pervasive muscle pain throughout the body)
- Headaches
- Musculoskeletal pain
- Myofascial pain (pain surrounding trigger points, or painful locations within muscles)
- Neuralgia (nerve disorder)

Healing the Pain

- Pain during childbirth
- Pain resulting from injury
- Pre- and postoperative pain
- Tinnitus (ringing or buzzing in the ears)

CAUTIONS IN USE OF TENS

Although the TENS technology is relatively simple, its use still demands vigilance. A few key cautions include:

- TENS should not be used on someone wearing a cardiac pacemaker because the TENS unit may disrupt proper functioning of the device.
- For patients with cardiac disorders, care must be taken that the TENS impulses don't have an adverse effect on heart rate.
- Pregnant women should not have electrodes attached to their abdomen.
- Electrodes should not be put on hypersensitive areas of the skin, on areas covered by a rash or lesions, or over an open wound.
- TENS electrodes should never be located over the carotid arteries (the major arteries on the neck that carry blood to the head) or over the muscles in the throat area.
- People with seizure or vascular disorders should not have the electrodes placed on their head or neck.
- TENS electrodes should never be placed near anyone's eyes.
- Burns can be an adverse effect of TENS if the unit isn't used

properly. For this reason, anyone with reduced skin sensitivity should avoid using TENS.

- Another side effect can be skin irritation. If it occurs, the electrodes should be changed or repositioned, or the transmitter settings may need to be adjusted. Electrodes should be removed regularly during prolonged treatments to avoid irritating the skin.

- The gel that is sometimes applied to electrode surfaces may cause an allergic reaction in some people.

- Painful muscle contractions can be another side effect, which can result in soreness and spasms. TENS should not be painful. If muscle contractions occur, it means the electrical impulse settings need adjusting.

- TENS should be used only with patients who are willing and able to play an active role in the treatment.

DOES TENS WORK?

Numerous studies supporting TENS as an effective pain-relief strategy appear in the medical literature as far back as the late 1960s. In recent years, however, the medical findings seem to be more mixed. Below is a sampling of results from recent studies:

TENS and osteoarthritis. Australian researchers, reporting in a 1994 issue of the *British Journal of Rheumatology*, compared TENS with naproxen (a nonsteroidal anti-inflammatory drug, or

NSAID) for treating 36 patients with osteoarthritis of the knee. One patient group received genuine naproxen plus placebo (or fake) TENS; another received a placebo drug plus genuine TENS, and a third received placebo forms of both the drug and TENS. The research team found no significant differences in pain relief among the three groups.

TENS and various pain syndromes. Reporting in a 1994 issue of *The Clinical Journal of Pain*, a group of Dutch researchers evaluated the effectiveness of TENS in more than 200 patients who had different pain disorders. Overall, 61 percent of the patients had enough pain relief after two to four weeks of treatment to want to continue with TENS. At the six-month follow-up point, 50 percent of the patients reported TENS was working for them.

Some types of pain responded better than others. The best success rates were found for angina (chest pain) from heart disease (75 percent), musculoskeletal problems due to degen-

---

Fish Came First

The use of electric current to alleviate pain can actually be traced back in time as far as the ancient Egyptians and Romans. They sent a mild charge into the body using electric fish, which were placed on the skin over a painful spot.

---

erative or mechanical causes (69 percent), and pain caused by peripheral nerve damage (53 percent). The researchers also found that about a third of the patients had some sort of side-effect, most commonly skin irritation. But any such problems were easily solved, usually by providing thorough instruction in how to use TENS.

TENS and painful menstruation. Swedish doctors compared TENS with naproxen in 12 women with dysmenorrhea, or painful menstruation. Before treatment, all of the women had uterine hyperactivity, causing increased pressure in the uterus. In an article in a 1994 issue of the *American Journal of Obstetrics and Gynecology*, the researchers reported that TENS brought some pain relief almost immediately, without changing uterine activity, and pain relief significantly increased after 30 to 60 minutes of treatment. In comparison, naproxen also eased the pain and suppressed uterine activity, but 19 to 120 minutes were needed for it to take effect.

TENS and acute low-back pain. A Canadian study published in *Spine* in 1994 followed a group of 58 industrial workers who had acute low back pain. The patients were divided into two groups: One participated in exercise and received genuine TENS, the other participated in exercise and received placebo TENS. The researchers found that exercise alone significantly reduced pain and disability. They found no added benefit from the TENS treatments.

A technological assessment of TENS. In a 1996 article in the *International Journal of Technology Assessment in Health Care*, Canadian researchers reviewed 79 English-language scientific articles published since 1974 on the effectiveness of TENS in treating acute or chronic pain. From their evaluation of the quality and findings of the studies, the research team concluded that although it is difficult to assess the effectiveness of TENS, "there is little evidence to recommend it."

SHOULD YOU TRY IT?

Despite some of the less convincing, or outright negative, reports on TENS, it remains in widespread use today. Even with the lack of sound scientific proof, many health practitioners and patients believe TENS is an effective treatment for pain.

Will it work for you? There's no way to predict, as individual responses vary widely. One of the key advantages to this technology is that it's easy and, except in very rare cases, painless to use. Given those factors, many people will continue to include TENS in the pain-fighting arsenal.

If you decide to try it, be sure you're under the guidance of a health practitioner who knows how to use TENS properly. Find out how much experience the practitioner has had with pain patients and whether any of those patients had painful conditions similar to yours.

CHAPTER 17
Conditions

You don't have to have a serious or life-threatening condition to experience severe pain. Common ailments such as arthritis and ear infection can also be accompanied by pain that is relentless. And you don't have to be in agony to need pain relief. Despite the bravery exhibited by actors in movies, there's no real value in stoically denying yourself medication or treatment that can make you more comfortable. In fact, research shows that keeping a stiff upper lip while you're experiencing pain can actually hurt you even more. Pain can interfere with recovery, lengthening the healing process.

Before you can treat your pain, however, you need to understand its cause. This chapter discusses 25 illnesses and conditions, all of which bring with them a variety of discomforts, including pain that runs the gamut from mild to debilitating. You'll learn the causes of each illness and how to treat the pain and discomfort it generates. When specific treatments are recommended, such as applying heat to ease arthritis pain, you can turn back to the chapter that covers that particular treatment for an in-depth discussion.

Finally, this section provides information about preventing these conditions and illnesses as well as the pain they can cause. Remember, prevention is your best defense against pain.

Arthritis

For most of us, the word *arthritis* conjures up an image of an older person with painful and swollen joints who can no longer do simple tasks, such as opening jars, fastening buttons, and lifting heavy grocery bags.

That image is only partly true, however. Actually, arthritis is an umbrella term for more than 100 different kinds of diseases, afflicting approximately one out of every seven Americans. Not all arthritis sufferers are elderly, and they don't all end up with the same disabilities.

Two Common Types

All arthritic conditions affect joints (the places where two bones and cartilage meet), muscle, and connective tissue. The two most common arthritic conditions are osteoarthritis and rheumatoid arthritis.

Osteoarthritis. This is the most prevalent form of arthritis, sometimes referred to as degenerative arthritis or "wear and tear" arthritis. Although traces of osteoarthritis may be seen in the X rays of people in their twenties and thirties, the disease rarely becomes a problem prior to age 45 and is more common among those age 65 and older. It starts with the breakdown of cartilage, the elastic tissue that lines and cushions the joints and allows bones to move smoothly against one another. When cartilage disintegrates, bone rubs on bone. The joint becomes misshapen and misaligned. Bony growths, called spurs, appear at the bone ends, and bits of loosened bone or cartilage may float around in the space surrounding the joint. These changes cause stiffness, swollen joints, and pain, especially in the knees, hips, fingers, spine, and feet.

Risk factors for osteoarthritis include the following: serious joint injury, consistent overuse of one or more joints, overweight, and a family history of osteoarthritis.

Rheumatoid arthritis. In this disease, inflammation sets in at the synovium, the thin membrane that lines and lubricates the joints. Inflammation causes swelling and pain, leading to erosion of bone and cartilage. Scar tissue gradually replaces the damaged cartilage, and the joint becomes rigid or misshapen and sometimes severely deformed. Rheumatoid arthritis affects connective tissue throughout the body and can adversely affect the heart, lungs, and eyes. Common accompanying conditions include anemia, fatigue, loss of appetite, muscle pain, weakness, and weight loss.

The inflammation of rheumatoid arthritis develops when the immune system attacks the body's own tissues. Medical researchers aren't sure what sets off this process. While various theories exist, research into causes continues. Meanwhile, it is hoped that research will also lead to new ways to control the disease.

The Variabilities of Arthritis

The discomfort and disability of arthritis can range from minor to severe. Even in one person, there are periods of remission—when there is relief from pain and other symptoms—and of flare-ups—when symptoms reappear, perhaps even more intensely than before.

Part of the challenge of arthritis is living with this uncertainty. The cycles of the disease also make it hard to know whether various treatments are effective. If you

Healing the Pain

begin to feel better, is it because you've hit upon an effective treatment, or is it just because you're in a remission phase?

What to Do for Arthritis

Getting a proper diagnosis is the first step in treating arthritis. If you've experienced joint stiffness and swelling that lasts for more than a couple of weeks, see a doctor for a physical examination to determine whether you have arthritis and, if so, what type it is.

Years ago, doctors advised people with arthritis to live a fairly sedentary life, resting a lot and exercising little. But no more. Modern research has shown that the proper balance between rest and exercise is crucial in treating arthritis. Too much exercise can exacerbate pain, especially during flare periods. But too little exercise weakens muscles, reduces joint mobility, and diminishes vitality. Exercise can also help trim excess weight, decreasing the load on your joints. It's important to get advice from a doctor or physical therapist about the right kind and intensity of exercise for your specific arthritis condition. And be sure the recommended exercises can be done at home.

For mild to moderate arthritis pain, over-the-counter medications can be effective. Aspirin and other NSAIDs (nonsteroidal anti-inflammatory drugs), such as ibuprofen and naproxen, help reduce the pain and swelling of rheumatoid arthritis. Many physicians suggest NSAIDs for osteoarthritis as well, but some research has shown that acetaminophen (Tylenol, for example) is just as effective. For more severe arthritis pain, your doctor may prescribe a stronger pain reliever. Some promising new treatments that suppress the over-active immune system have recently become available by prescription for those with rheumatoid arthritis. Again, ask your doctor to see if this might be appropriate for you.

Heat, in such forms as a hot compress, a heating pad, or warm whirlpool bath, can also ease arthritis pain, as can a topical cream containing capsaicin, the chemical found in hot chili peppers. Some people find cold treatments, such as ice packs or soaking a joint in cold water, a better way to relieve arthritis pain, especially when there is swelling. Or you can alternate heat and cold. For example, soak the affected body part in warm water for three minutes, then soak in cold water for a minute. Repeat three times, ending with a soak in warm water.

Back Pain

Odds are you won't escape having at least one episode of back pain in your lifetime. Statistics show that back pain strikes four out of five people. Most pain of this sort centers in the lower back, near the inward curve of the back and just above the base of the spine—the area that carries the majority of our weight.

When our back hurts, the first question we usually ask is: What on earth did I do to cause such pain? Sometimes we can pinpoint a specific action, such as lifting a heavy box or twisting the wrong way, but often we're not sure of the cause.

The fact that humans rely on only two legs to support our bodies has much to do with our tendency to have back problems. Other mammals are supported by four legs as they move about. Human backs, then, are under much more stress.

Causes

Back pain can be triggered by a number of diverse conditions, including:

- Osteoarthritis of the spine (see the section on arthritis)
- Herniated disk, which inflames ligaments and causes muscle spasm around the spine
- Stress or anxiety with preexisting minor back problems
- Pregnancy, due to the additional bodyweight and altered weight distribution brought on by the pregnancy or the position of the fetus, or both
- Menstruation
- Overweight
- Osteoporosis
- Fibromyalgia (see the section on fibromyalgia)

In many cases, however, back pain simply arises from sprains and strains of muscles and ligaments. Studies show that more than 90 percent of the problems associated with back pain disappear on their own, usually within four weeks, but almost always within six weeks.

If you have a backache that lasts more than a week or two, see a doctor to rule out possible serious conditions, such as disorders of the bones, intestinal tract, kidneys, lungs, or reproductive organs. If your back pain is accompanied by the following symptoms, see your doctor without delay:

- loss of bladder or bowel control
- weakness or numbness in the rectal or groin area
- weakness or numbness in the arms, legs, or feet
- progressive weakness or numbness in one extremity—such as

Healing the Pain

being unable to move a toe one day, the whole foot the next

- fever
- loss of muscle control
- personal history of cancer
- unexplained weight loss
- pain that shoots down the leg into the calf
- back pain resulting from a fall or blow to the back
- back pain that's getting worse
- back pain that's worse when lying down or that's much worse at night than in the daytime
- back pain in someone younger than 20 years of age

Prevention

Back pain is a common affliction, but you're not necessarily doomed to recurring bouts of it. Take these steps to diminish your risks:

Build a strong back. Most doctors think exercise is the crucial ingredient in back pain prevention. It helps you shed extra pounds, and it strengthens the muscles that support the back (including the abdominal muscles).

Maintain good posture. Slumping and slouching while standing or sitting will strain your back. As you go about daily activities, notice if you're maintaining the back's normal curvature. Sometimes using a simple device can help—such as placing a pillow behind the small of your back when you're sitting. If you're prone to back problems, the best sleeping position is either on your side, with your knees bent and a pillow between them, or on your back, with a pillow placed under your knees.

Lift right. Lift heavy objects by bending your knees and putting your arms at the same level as the object you're about to lift. Use your legs, not your back, to power your lift. Keep your back straight.

Stop smoking. Smoking affects more than the lungs and heart. Studies show smokers are more likely to have back problems.

Lose weight. To decrease the load your back has to support, shed a few pounds.

What to Do for Back Pain

When you're plagued with back pain, you may need to rest for a couple of days at first, depending on the severity of the pain. But don't sit or lie around for long. You'll just make matters worse by losing muscle tone, which can mean more back trouble in the future. Get up and about as soon as you can. As you become active, you can use lower back braces and supporting belts to relieve pain and provide support. But most doctors advise wearing these only for short periods or during back-straining activities; otherwise these supporting devices can result in weakened muscles.

Many medical studies have shown that exercising to build up weak muscles is a basic part of back care, both for healing back pain and for preventing future problems. If you're in the midst of a back-pain episode, check with your health practitioner before starting an exercise program. The wrong kind of exercise could make the pain worse. Gentle, nonjarring exercises are best. If you've had back problems in the past or have a major health condition, such as osteoporosis, checking with your doctor before starting exercise is crucial.

A physical therapist can help you get off to a safe start. A complete exercise program should include a warm-up period followed by stretching, strengthening exercises, a cool-down period, and more stretching.

Chiropractic is another treatment technique that reportedly works well for back pain. A chiropractor manipulates the spine to try to relieve subluxations, or misalignments in the spine, that can put pressure on nerves. According to chiropractic theory, the health of the nervous system is restored and the body's natural healing processes can take effect when there are no misalignments in the spine.

Many back-pain sufferers find that a massage is a great way to relieve back pain. Exactly how massage works is unclear. Some believe that pressure applied during massage prevents pain signals from getting through to the brain. Others believe that massage reduces pain by curbing the body's production of stress hormones and enhancing the flow of natural painkillers. Massage also relaxes tense muscles and stimulates blood circulation.

Heat or cold can be therapeutic for back pain, although there is disagreement in the medical community as to which is more effective. While heat has been the traditional treatment, some doctors claim that applying cold, such as by rubbing the painful area with an ice pack, works better. Still, some people are more comfortable applying heat. Experiment with both to see which works best for your pain.

Bursitis

Throughout the body there are some 150 fluid-filled sacs that cushion the muscles and ligaments around your joints, where two or more bones meet. Called bursae (plural for bursa), these sacs contain a lubricating fluid that eliminates friction and allows the tendons and muscles in your joint areas to move smoothly.

Healing the Pain

Bursitis, a condition characterized by tenderness and swelling near a joint area, is caused by inflammation of a bursa. The most common joint affected is the shoulder, but bursitis can strike almost any joint. In severe cases, swelling and calcium deposits can make joint movement impossible.

The inflammation of a bursa can result from constant, repetitive use of certain joints or from excessive pressure on them. But it can also develop suddenly, as from a sports injury or other abrupt body stress. And it can be the result of an activity you're not used to doing or from a more intense session of one of your usual activities—such as increasing your usual jogging distance from six miles to ten or walking at a faster pace.

In still other cases, you may have no idea what you did to trigger the bursitis.

Bursitis also can coexist with other conditions, such as arthritis, making it difficult to know which one is causing pain at a particular time. Thus, people who have arthritis shouldn't necessarily assume that worsened joint pain is just their arthritis acting up. See your doctor if you are unsure of the reason for any joint pain.

Prevention

If you've had bursitis in the past, you can take steps to ward off another occurrence:

- Build up your muscles. Keeping muscles toned protects joints.
- Use padding. Prolonged or excessive pressure on joints can increase the chances for bursitis. Sit in a cushioned chair if you spend hours at a desk job. Or put a foam pad under your knees when you scrub the floor.
- Break up repetitive tasks. If you're doing the same sort of

motion over and over all day, make it easier on your joints by switching to a different activity now and then.

- Ease up. Be aware of when you're putting excessive stress and pressure on your joints, and give them a rest.

What to Do for Bursitis

During a bout of bursitis, be extra careful not to put pressure on the sore joint area. At first you may need to use a sling, elastic bandage, or crutches to relieve the affected joint until the inflammation lessens.

At the same time, you don't want to keep the joint immobilized any longer than necessary, or you'll risk reducing your normal range of motion. Just move prudently to protect the sensitive joint, and be sure to avoid whatever activity set off the bursitis in the first place.

If the pain doesn't get much better after a few days, see your doctor to determine if the cause of your pain is something other than bursitis.

To alleviate pain and inflammation, take nonprescription NSAIDs (nonsteroidal anti-inflammatory drugs), such as ibuprofen or naproxen. If necessary, your doctor may give you an injection of a corticosteroid in the affected area.

Ice packs placed over the affected joint will also reduce pain and inflammation. Once the tenderness and swelling have diminished (usually within a few days), a heating pad or hot compress—or perhaps alternating hot and cold compresses—may make you more comfortable during the healing process.

Acupuncture may also ease the pain and swelling of bursitis. In addition to inserting thin needles

Healing the Pain

at meridian points (see the chapter on acupuncture), the acupuncturist may prescribe herbal treatments.

Cancer Pain

Cancer is one of the most feared diagnoses. But it is no longer necessarily a death sentence. As detection and treatment methods improve, more and more cancer patients survive. And many of those who do not respond as well to treatment are at least able to enjoy a longer and more productive life than would have been possible some years ago.

Still, for millions of people fighting cancer, a trying, exhausting, and frightening aspect of the battle is enduring the pain. Cancer pain can be physically debilitating—often causing poor sleep, appetite loss, and other negative physical effects—and emotionally devastating. For cancer patients, the pain is a constant reminder of how sick they are and a foreboding of an uncertain future. As a result, anxiety and depression can easily set in.

Many different factors can cause cancer pain. Often it's the result of a tumor pressing on a bone, organ, or nerve. Chemotherapy, surgery, and other cancer therapies can also cause pain during and after the procedure.

What can and should be done to relieve cancer pain? That question has been the focus of much debate in medical circles in recent years. Research has revealed a wide variance in how cancer patients are treated for pain. Whether a particular patient gets adequate relief often depends on how much his or her doctor knows about pain control.

Healing the Pain

Medical experts say that, in general, pain caused by cancer is dramatically undertreated. Yet they point out that adequate pain relief can be achieved in 90 percent of cancer cases. This discrepancy between what is done and what could be done spurred the Agency for Health Care Policy and Research (AHCPR) of the U.S. Department of Health and Human Services to set up an expert panel in 1991 to study the problem.

Attitudes That Obstruct Cancer Pain Control

The AHCPR panel cited several common beliefs—often shared by doctors and health consumers—that prevent patients from receiving the pain treatment they need. Among these are the following:

- "Pain is an inevitable and untreatable consequence of cancer." On the contrary, the panel stressed that almost all cancer pain can be controlled.

- "Reporting pain is a weakness." Some people don't want to complain, feeling they'll come across as troublesome patients. But they need to feel free to discuss their pain and tell doctors when pain treatments are working and when they're not.

- "Pain medication is addictive." Practitioners and patients alike fear that using opioids (such as morphine) for more severe cancer pain will lead to addiction. But there is a distinction between addiction and dependence. (For more on this subject see the chapter on prescription medications.)

- "Using a medication early means it won't work later." People sometimes believe medication should be "saved" for later when the pain is expected to worsen. But early pain relief is crucial, before pain takes a firm hold and becomes more difficult to treat.

Healing the Pain

Moreover, pain treatment won't stop working over time if appropriate adjustments are made in dosages or in types of medication needed.

- "The side effects are worse than the pain." Some people will put up with pain because of apprehensions about side effects. But there are many different types of pain medication. If one causes side effects in a particular patient, another may not. Or perhaps an alternative or additional treatment can counter the side effects and still bring pain relief.

What to Do for Cancer Pain

A major message that came out of the AHCPR panel's work was that much more could be done to relieve the pain of cancer patients. After reviewing more than 9,600 published resources and consulting hundreds of outside experts, the panel issued its clinical practice guidelines in 1994. The purpose of the guidelines is to better inform practicing physicians about what can and should be done to help people cope with cancer pain. Health care consumers can also use this information to be sure their doctors are doing everything possible to alleviate cancer pain.

Below is a sampling of some of the panel's key recommendations.

- Pain treatment should begin early and be aggressive in order to prevent unnecessary suffering.
- Effective treatment begins with pain assessment, relying heavily on patient input. For children, the elderly, or others who have difficulty communicating verbally, nonverbal assessment techniques, such as pictorial representations and studying the patient's behavior, can be used.
- Drug therapy is the cornerstone of cancer pain management and

should be based on the needs of the patient. The least invasive treatment—such as medication administered orally rather than in the form of injection—should be tried first.

- For mild cancer pain, NSAIDs (nonsteroidal anti-inflammatory drugs) such as aspirin and ibuprofen may provide adequate relief.

- Opioids, such as morphine, may be needed for severe types of cancer pain. The panel emphasized the difference between physical dependence and addiction. While long-term opioid use may cause physical dependence, it does not cause addiction, which is a person's compulsive need to use a drug. (For more information, see the chapter on prescription medications.)

- Physical treatments can help patients cope with pain, but should not substitute for medication. Treatments may include exercise, heat, cold, massage, transcutaneous electrical nerve stimulation (TENS), and acupuncture. The panel recommended that patients should undergo acupuncture only after reporting any new pain to the doctor, since this could be an indicator of the course of the disease.

- Psychosocial interventions may also play an important part in pain management (again, not as a substitute for medications). Relaxation techniques, guided imagery, cognitive restructuring, support groups, and pastoral care were among the techniques the panel felt had proved effective.

- Invasive interventions, such as radiation therapy, nerve blocks, and surgery may be needed when other treatments aren't successful.

Healing the Pain

Carpal Tunnel Syndrome

Carpal tunnel syndrome (CTS) has become the plague of the computer generation. But it isn't just people who punch computer keys all day who develop the condition, which is also known by a variety of other names, including repetitive motion injury. Those who spend a great deal of time every day with their wrists flexed or in extended positions—especially if they also do a lot of repeated grasping, twisting, turning, or pinching with the hands or wrist—are at increased risk for CTS. Typists, assembly-line workers, and cashiers, for example, are prime candidates for CTS.

Pressure and vibration can also trigger the condition, making people who spend hours operating jackhammers and electric drills susceptible to the syndrome. But CTS doesn't have to be related to on-the-job activities. Even hobbies, such as knitting and playing video games, involve the kind of movements that set the stage for CTS.

Pain is the dominant symptom of CTS, but there may also be weakness, numbness, tingling, burning, swelling, and stiffness. These sensations can be felt in the palm, thumb, and the first three fingers of the hand, or back toward the elbow. CTS may occur in both hands at the same time or in only one hand. The pain and other symptoms may be constant or intermittent; they are often worse during or shortly after the activity that triggered the syndrome.

Accurate Diagnosis Is Crucial

The carpal tunnel is formed by the bones of the wrist and the tough band of connective tissue known as the transverse carpal ligament. Inside this tunnel lie the median nerve and the tendons used to bend the fingers and thumb. When the tissue lining the inside of the carpal tunnel swells, it puts pressure on the median nerve, and that sets off the CTS symptoms.

In addition, certain health conditions can also trigger CTS. For instance, pregnancy can bring on generalized swelling of body tissues, including the carpal tunnel. Hypothyroidism (low levels of the thyroid hormone) and diabetes may cause CTS symptoms, as can rheumatoid arthritis, obesity, and smoking. Treating these problems may in itself alleviate CTS. On the other hand, symptoms that suggest CTS may instead be signs of a wrist fracture, sprain, dislocation, benign tumor, or various other medical conditions.

It's critical to determine the cause of CTS in order to receive appropriate treatment. Simply guessing that you have CTS because your symptoms are "just like Jane's who works at the next desk" is not good enough. Nor is adopting Jane's approach to treatment because it worked for her. See a doctor to find out whether you actually have CTS or if you have some other condition that needs to be treated first. Remember, if you ignore CTS, you can cause long-term damage that can even be permanent.

What to Do for Carpal Tunnel Syndrome

If you have a job or hobby that involves repetitive movements, you can reduce your risks of CTS—or avoid worsening the condition if you already have it— by taking frequent breaks. Stop for a couple of minutes every half hour, with a slightly longer break after an hour. And switch tasks occasionally to avoid repeating the same kind of motion.

During your break time, try the following simple hand and wrist exercises. But if they cause increased pain, stop them immediately and make an appointment to see your doctor.

- Hold your hands out in front of you, palms down, parallel to the floor. Keep your wrists steady while you rotate your hands in circles, both clockwise and counterclockwise.
- Spread your fingers and thumb out far apart and hold for a few seconds.
- Tightly squeeze a small rubber ball in your hand five to ten times, then stretch out your fingers.

While involved in any daily activity, pay attention to your body posi-

tion. Wrists should be in a neutral position—that is, in a straight line with your forearms, not bent up or down. Your computer keyboard should be at a height that allows this neutral position. Your computer screen should be just below eye level to prevent body strain.

Notice how you grip objects with your hands. If you're opening a jar, for instance, you should grasp the lid with your whole hand, not just with your thumb and first two fingers, as that puts more pressure on one side of the wrist. Fortunately, many power tools today are made to vibrate less than older models, so it is not necessary to hold them as tightly as before. Also, be sure that tools aren't too large for your hand, so your hand isn't forced into an awkward position while holding them.

Staying in shape, keeping your weight down, and avoiding smok-

Healing the Pain

ing also can prevent CTS or keep it from getting worse.

If you have CTS, your doctor may suggest that you wear a splint to immobilize the wrist and keep the symptoms from getting worse. Some people tend to tuck their hands under their head at night with their wrists bent. This position aggravates CTS. Wearing a splint while sleeping can help keep your wrists in a neutral position.

Taking over-the-counter NSAIDs (ibuprofen and others) can help relieve CTS pain. Some recent research has shown that vitamin B_6 supplementation reduces symptoms, although more evidence is needed to verify this finding. Note that high doses of this vitamin can be toxic, so be sure to consult a health professional about its use.

If the preceding measures fail to eliminate or reduce your pain,

consult a physician. Injections of a local anesthetic and corticosteroids may bring the pain under control.

Surgery to cut open the ligament covering the carpal tunnel has also been shown to be an effective treatment for CTS.

Chest Pain

Chest pain can be a symptom of many health problems, ranging from indigestion to a heart attack. The natural tendency is to write the chest pain off as "just something I ate." But whenever you have serious chest pain, it's best to let a doctor determine if your pain is minor, major, or something in between.

Causes

The following are a few health conditions that might bring on chest pain, along with some clues to help differentiate one from another.

Indigestion and heartburn. A burning or gnawing sensation in the chest, or feelings of pressure, could be a sign of digestive troubles. Sometimes it's easy to mistake this kind of pain for angina (see below). But pain associated with digestive problems usually will get worse when you lie down.

Heartburn results when stomach acid migrates up into the lower portion of the esophagus (the tube connecting the mouth to the stomach). The lower esophageal sphincter is a muscle that's supposed to keep stomach acid in your stomach. If it becomes weakened or abnormally relaxed, the sphincter can open, allowing upward movement of stomach acid. Being overweight can weaken the sphincter, and ingesting certain substances—such as alcohol, caffeine, chocolate, and nicotine—can cause it to relax. Simply eating too much or lying down after a meal can also trigger heartburn.

Pleurisy. This is an inflammation of the pleura, the membrane surrounding the lungs and lining the chest cavity. The pain of pleurisy can be sharp and stabbing, or just plain uncomfortable. It's usually felt on one side of the chest and may diminish when you sit up. Coughing, sneezing, swallowing, and deep breathing may make the pain worse.

Angina pectoris. In this condition, some part of the heart muscle does not get enough blood and, therefore, does not get enough of the oxygen carried by the blood. An angina attack is not a heart attack, however. Heart muscle isn't necessarily damaged in angina, as it is by a heart attack. The most common cause of angina is atherosclerosis (narrowing of the arteries due to fatty deposits).

Angina pain is often described as dull and constricting and is usually located in the center of the chest beneath the breastbone. It may feel like pressure, squeezing, or burning, and it can closely resemble indigestion or heartburn. The pain may radiate to the arms, shoulders (usually the left one), neck, jaws, or back. An angina attack usually lasts no more than five minutes, and resting or taking nitroglycerin reduces the pain.

Heart attack. A heart attack (also known technically as a myocardial infarction, or MI) results in pain that is similar to the pain of angina, but it is usually more severe and longer lasting. It feels like a heavy pressure, constriction, or burning sensation beneath the breastbone. The pain may radiate to the arms (usually the left one), neck, jaw, or back. Other symptoms include extreme anxiety, nausea, paleness, restlessness, sweating, and vomiting. Neither rest nor nitroglycerin reduces the pain of heart attack.

Anxiety. Just as chest pain can produce anxiety, so can anxiety be the cause of chest pain. It can be mild to severe and may feel dull, heavy, or sharp. A choking sensation, dry mouth, palpitations, nausea, shortness of breath, sweating, and trembling may be accompanying symptoms. Rest and relaxation help alleviate the symptoms.

Other conditions. Several chest, heart, lung, and other health conditions may also have chest pain as a major symptom.

What to Do for Chest Pain

The best thing you can do for serious chest pain is to see your doctor. Waiting too long to get the treatment you need could endanger your life.

Healing the Pain

If heartburn is the cause of your chest pain, you can probably relieve the discomfort by taking over-the-counter antacids. If you prefer an herbal alternative, try ginger, freshly ground from gingerroot. Teas made from gentian root, dandelion root, wormwood, goldenseal root, fennel seeds, lemon balm leaves, and peppermint leaves also have a soothing effect. These herbal remedies reportedly serve as preventative measures as well.

Be sure to avoid foods that set off your heartburn, whether they be fatty foods, hot spices, chocolate, coffee, or other substances, and avoid eating just before lying down. Being overweight also increases your chances of developing heartburn.

If your chest pain is due to angina pectoris, your doctor may recommend lifestyle changes, such as getting proper exercise, modifying your diet, reaching and maintaining a healthy weight, or stopping smoking. Stress-reduction methods, such as biofeedback, imagery, and meditation, may also be useful. Many doctors recommend taking aspirin on a regular basis, but be sure to check with your doctor to see if it is appropriate before considering such a program for yourself. Prescription medications that increase the blood flow to the heart, such as nitroglycerin, commonly are part of angina treatment. Other preventive medications include calcium antagonists, which block constriction of arterial muscles, and beta blockers, which slow the heart's activity level and therefore reduce its demand for oxygen.

For angina pain, a practitioner of herbal medicine might recommend an extract of hawthorn berries, which are said to relieve chest pain by widening coronary arteries and allowing more blood to get to the heart muscle. Don't forget to tell your physician if you intend to take herbal medications.

Dental Pain

For many of us, just thinking about going to the dentist is enough to make us uncomfortable. No one relishes the thought of having cavities drilled, teeth extracted, or a root canal procedure. Yet pain in our teeth or jaw will drive us to the dentist in the hope of finding relief.

Causes

Dental pain can have various causes, including:

Tooth decay. When decay progresses into the dentin (the bony second layer under your tooth enamel) or into the surface of an exposed root, you will feel pain. Your tooth may be sensitive to touch or to sudden changes in temperature, or both. And if bacteria pass through tiny channels in the dentin and then into the tooth pulp, where the blood vessels and nerve tissue are located, you'll end up with a dandy toothache.

Periodontal disease. This condition consists of progressive deterioration of the gums, bones, and other tissues around the teeth. In the early stages of periodontal disease, gums are sore, red, and slightly swollen. They may be sensitive to the touch and bleed when brushed or flossed. The second stage of this disease is marked by pus in the gums around the teeth, which can cause swelling and extreme pain.

Other problems. Sometimes tooth pain is one symptom, among others, of some specific condition,

Healing the Pain

such as temporomandibular disorders (TMD). (See separate section on TMD.)

What to Do for Dental Pain

The first step in treating dental pain is finding out what's causing it. If something in your mouth or jaw hurts, it's best to pay a visit to your dentist.

Mild pain that comes in the aftermath of dental work can usually be treated with over-the-counter pain-relieving medications. For more severe pain, such as that which often accompanies the extraction of wisdom teeth as well as other surgical procedures, the dentist may prescribe a stronger painkiller, such as an opioid like codeine.

As for alleviating pain that is caused during a dental procedure, dentists often turn to an anesthetic such as Novocain. Although the shot itself can be painful, anesthetic injections help us get through the dentist's drilling without feeling pain.

Innovations in dental anesthesia may someday make visits to the dentist much more tolerable. One of these is the dental patch, currently undergoing trials for the Food and Drug Administration. The patch contains a pain-killing substance and has a special gummed backing that adheres to the mucous membranes of the mouth. When and if the patch comes into widespread use, it probably will serve mostly as a pre-injection anesthetic to numb the skin at the injection site. This will be a welcome development for people who detest Novocain shots. The patch could also be used to relieve pain from mouth sores and lesions.

Electronic dental anesthesia using transcutaneous electrical nerve stimulation (TENS) may be another wave of the future. Actually, electronic anesthesia is not new in dentistry. But only recently have reliable, less expensive devices been developed, and now they are more widely available in dentists' offices.

TENS anesthesia involves attaching electrodes outside your mouth, near the area to be worked on. An electric current, controlled by the patient or dentist, is transmitted through the electrodes to the nerves in your mouth. These electric impulses block pain signals traveling from your mouth to your brain.

As more research is done and this technology continues to improve, many dentists believe TENS anesthesia will see increased application in dentistry in the future. It may be used for such routine procedures as filling cavities and eas-

ing the pain of injections rather than for tooth extractions and other more painful procedures.

Ear Pain

We rarely pay much attention to our ears—until we feel pain in them. Then it's hard not to notice them. Several conditions can cause ear pain; the following are a few of the most common ones.

Injury or Trauma

A sharp blow to the side of the head or exposure to a particularly loud noise, such as an explosion, can result in injuries inside the ear, such as a ruptured or perforated eardrum. (The eardrum is the thin membrane that separates the outer ear from the middle ear.)

Another common way people damage their eardrums is by putting objects such as bobby pins or cotton-tipped swabs in their ear in an effort to clean out wax or relieve itching. Doing so may have the unintended result of pushing wax up against the eardrum, reducing its ability to vibrate and transmit sound waves; it could even puncture the eardrum.

Swimmer's Ear

Swimmer's ear can result when fungus or bacteria nestle into an outer ear canal that is warm and moist. There the fungus or bacteria thrive. Frequent exposure to water creates such conditions (hence the name) and also washes away the oily, waxy substance that naturally lines the ear canal and protects against infection.

But swimming isn't the only activity that can set the scene for an outer-ear infection. It's fairly common in any warm, humid climate. Nor is moisture the only culprit. Poking around in the outer ear canal with an object, including a cotton-tipped swab, can scratch the delicate lining of the ear canal and break down the natural barriers against infection.

No matter what triggers it, swimmer's ear starts with an itching or tingling in the ear. Severe cases can lead to pain and discharge or even some hearing loss because of swelling in the outer-ear canal.

Blocked Eustachian Tube

The eustachian tube is a thin, membrane-lined tube connecting the middle ear with the back of the nose and throat. When this tube remains clear, the air pressure on both sides of the eardrum stays roughly equal. If something blocks the eustachian tube, however, the air supply doesn't get to the middle ear, and this creates a vacuum. The eardrum gets sucked inward, stretching it taut and sometimes causing pain.

If you have ever traveled by airplane when you had a stuffed nose, you may have experienced this sensation. During take-off and landing, air pressure in the plane's cabin falls and rises rapidly. Normally the air inside the middle ear would equalize on its own, but not if congestion is blocking the eustachian tube.

Tinnitus

Tinnitus is a ringing or buzzing in the ears that results when the tiny hair cells in the inner ear become damaged. These hair cells normally pick up sound vibrations and send electrical impulses through the auditory nerve to the brain. In tinnitus, the hair cells are "on" all the time, and the brain thinks sounds are entering the ear nonstop.

Loud noise, ear wax, ear infection, a perforated eardrum, fluid accumulation in the ear, high blood pressure, allergies, a tumor, thyroid problems, diabetes, and normal aging processes are just some of the causes of tinnitus.

Middle-ear Infection

Middle-ear infection, or otitis media by its medical name, can strike anyone of any age, but it especially plagues children of preschool age. Nearly 70 percent of children in the United States have at least one ear infection by their second birthday. Overall, it's the second most common illness among U.S. children, ranking after the common cold. Of even greater concern is the fact that middle-ear infections are becoming more frequent. Statistics from the Centers for Disease Control and Prevention show that doctors' visits for middle-ear infections jumped 150 percent from 1975 to 1990.

Most often a middle-ear infection sets in when a child has a cold. Bacteria can travel up the eustachian tube into the middle ear. As the infection develops, pus builds up, creating pressure in the middle ear that leads to pain. Young children are more prone to such infections than adults because their eustachian tubes are shorter and at such an angle that it's easier for bacteria to back up from the nose to the middle ear.

Symptoms of middle-ear infection include crying, fussiness, fever, nausea, and vomiting. Young children who have a middle-ear infection may indicate discomfort by repeatedly tugging on their ears.

Sometimes fluid accumulates and thickens in the middle ear, even when no infection exists. This condition is known as otitis media with effusion, also known as "glue ear." The child may have no pain, but you may notice signs of hearing loss that are caused by the fluid build-up.

What to Do for Ear Pain

Here are some strategies for preventing and treating each of the types of ear problems just described.

Ear injury or trauma. Follow the old folk wisdom about never putting anything smaller than an elbow into your ear. If, despite this advice, you sustain an injury or trauma and suspect eardrum damage, see a doctor. Never try to treat an ear injury yourself.

Swimmer's ear. To prevent this condition, be sure to shake all the water out of your ears after swimming or showering. If your efforts at prevention fail, over-the-counter eardrops may relieve the symptoms, or you can make a home remedy consisting of equal parts rubbing alcohol and white vinegar. Before using any kind of eardrops, however, check with your doctor, especially if you have had eardrum damage. See your doctor in cases of serious pain or discharge. Finally, never poke around in your ear with swabs or other objects to relieve itching.

Blocked eustachian tubes. Swallowing, yawning, and chewing gum are normally enough to equalize the pressure in your middle ear and prevent or relieve pain. If you must fly while you have a cold, try a decongestant to help keep your eustachian tubes open.

Tinnitus. Stay away from loud noises if possible; wear ear protection if you cannot escape from a noisy environment. Avoid caffeine and tobacco, which can spark tinnitus. If the condition persists and you're not sure of the cause, see your doctor to rule out a serious underlying health problem.

Middle-ear infection. One key preventive measure is to avoid exposing children to cigarette smoke, which boosts the risk of middle-ear infection. And try as much as possible to keep your son or daughter away from other children who are sick. For infants, another preventive step may be breast-feeding, which helps them build resistance to ear infections. Finally, babies shouldn't fall asleep while taking fluid from a bottle, since the fluid could seep into their eustachian tubes.

To treat middle-ear infections, many doctors prescribe an antibiotic, though much disagreement exists in the medical community about this practice. Many physicians feel it's the best course of treatment; others claim that the overuse of antibiotics leads to resistant bacterial strains and thus to ever-growing problems in treating middle-ear infections.

Chiropractors believe that manipulations of the neck or base of the

Healing the Pain

skull offer promise to adults and children who are bothered with an infection of the ear.

⁂

Endometriosis

Endometriosis is a condition affecting females that continues to challenge medical experts, though researchers may be getting closer to a solution. This disease can be difficult to diagnose accurately, and some women go through years of pain before they find out that they have it. Exact causes are unknown. Recent research suggests a possible connection to exposure to the environmental pollutant dioxin, but even if this connection is supported by future studies, it would explain only a small percentage of cases. According to the Milwaukee-based Endometriosis Association, about five million women in the U.S. have the disease. Of that number, 41 percent say they first had symptoms in their teens, and some were as young as age 11 at onset.

In endometriosis, fragments of the uterine lining become implanted outside the uterus, usually somewhere else in the abdominal cavity. Exactly how these fragments get to other parts of the body remains unclear. At any rate, these implants respond to hormonal changes in a woman's body just as they would if they were part of the uterine lining that gets sloughed off each month during menstruation. Because these implants are outside the uterus, however, the blood flowing from them has no way to exit the body and so becomes absorbed by surrounding tissue. This can result in pain. As the months go on, the implants may grow and multiply, sometimes forming scar tissue or blood-filled sacs or cysts. If a cyst bursts, the resulting pain can be severe.

Symptoms vary greatly. Some women have little or no pain; for others the pain is excruciating. Some pain starts when menstruation begins, which may be why endometriosis so often remains undiagnosed: Women figure it's just part of the menstrual discomfort they have to endure. In other women, the pain begins at different points of their monthly cycle. If the endometrial implants affect a woman's bladder or intestines, she also may experience painful urination or bowel movements and perhaps blood in the urine or stools. Other symptoms may include premenstrual staining and excessive menstrual blood flow.

Research shows a link between endometriosis and infertility; 30 to 40 percent of infertile women are also troubled by endometriosis. Still, medical experts don't know for sure which condition causes the other, if indeed there is a causal relationship.

The only way a doctor can make a definite diagnosis of endometriosis is by a procedure called laparoscopy, in which a tubelike instrument is inserted into the lower abdomen through a tiny incision. This device allows the doctor to look at the displaced tissue. A laparoscopy requires anesthesia, but it usually doesn't necessitate an overnight stay in the hospital.

What to Do for Endometriosis

All too often in the past, endometriosis went undiagnosed until a woman's pain was so severe and her symptoms so advanced that she had to undergo surgery to remove the uterus (a hysterectomy) and the ovaries (an oophorectomy). But today, with early diagnosis and treatment, such drastic measures are not often needed. That's why it's important for women—even young teens—who experience severe pain to not simply assume that it's "just my period." Diagnosis of endometriosis in its early stages boosts the chances of controlling the disease before it gets worse.

Although doctors can't cure endometriosis, they can treat the symptoms and usually relieve the pain. Three key medications now in use include:

- Danazol. This is a synthetic hormone that shrinks the endometrial implants. It is expensive, however, and possible side effects include weight gain, facial hair, and deepened voice.
- Nasal spray containing nafarelin acetate. This is used to shrink implants and relieve symptoms. Side effects such as hot flashes and vaginal dryness mimic symptoms of menopause.
- Injections of leuprolide acetate. Monthly injections for six months relieve symptoms and have the same side effects as the nasal spray described above.

If medication proves unsuccessful, surgery may be necessary. Today doctors can perform laser surgery with the aid of a laparoscope, the instrument described earlier. A carefully focused laser beam can destroy the endometrial tissue. This procedure usually can be done without having to spend the night in the hospital, and only about one week's recovery time will be needed at home.

When neither medication nor conservative surgery relieves symptoms of endometriosis, removal of the uterus and ovaries may be the next step.

A pain clinic may also offer help for some women who suffer from endometriosis. For example, a woman who wants to have children would be reluctant to agree to having her uterus removed and would require an optional form of treatment. But even women who consent to a hysterectomy may still experience continued pain. In either case, pain clinics offer treatment that may help reduce the pain and suffering, allowing women to return to a more normal lifestyle.

Those wishing to try an alternative approach might consider acupuncture, which involves insertion and manipulation of fine needles to stimulate life energy. In the Oriental view, a condition such as endometriosis results when the body's energy, or qi (pronounced "chee"), is out of balance. Acupuncture aims to restore balance and, thus, health. Usually, the acupuncturist will also prescribe herbal medicines to augment the acupuncture treatments.

Fibroid Tumors

As ominous as the term "fibroid tumors" may sound, this condition is actually quite common among women and is almost never life threatening. Statistics show that as many as 40 percent of women have fibroids by the time they reach age 40. The rate of occurrence is highest among black women.

A fibroid tumor is a mass of muscle and connective tissue that can grow inside the uterine wall, from the uterine wall extending out into the abdominal cavity, or from the uterine wall inward into the uterus itself. Fibroids can range in size from minuscule to several

Healing the Pain

inches in diameter. Although it's possible to have a single fibroid, it's more common for them to show up in numbers. In the vast majority of cases, these growths are benign, with less than one percent ever becoming cancerous.

Still, even though benign, fibroids can cause uncomfortable symptoms. Some women find their periods last longer than usual, with heavier bleeding. In severe cases, the extra blood loss can lead to anemia or an abnormally low level of red blood cells. Sometimes fibroids press against the bladder, triggering the desire to urinate more frequently. Pressure on the ureters (the tubes connecting the bladder to the kidneys) can lead to urinary tract and kidney infections, while pressure on the bowels may cause constipation. Another symptom is pelvic pain and a feeling of heaviness in the pelvic region.

Sometimes a woman's abdomen will protrude, making her look as if she's in the early stages of pregnancy. Fibroids can also result in infertility and miscarriage, or they may cause complications during pregnancy as the fetus grows.

Still, many women remain symptom free or experience only mild symptoms, even when their fibroids are quite large. Often a woman won't know she has fibroid tumors until her doctor discovers them during a routine pelvic examination.

Doctors aren't sure what causes fibroids, although estrogen apparently plays a part in their development. That's not to say that estrogen causes fibroids, but rather that estrogen stimulates their growth. At menopause, when estrogen production drops off, fibroids begin to shrink and, perhaps, eventually disappear.

What to Do
for Fibroid Tumors

Until recently, the common rule of thumb was that when fibroids grew big enough so that the uterus became as large as if in the twelfth week of pregnancy, then a hysterectomy (removal of the uterus) was in order—even if a woman was symptom free. The thinking was that surgery should be done before the fibroids grew any larger and thus became more difficult to remove.

Now many doctors argue against this approach, choosing instead to simply monitor fibroids. As long as a woman has no serious problems, according to these medical experts, no treatment of any kind is necessary. Other doctors continue to advise hysterectomies for fibroids, which account for about 30 percent of the more than half-million hysterectomies performed annually in the United States.

If and when a fibroid condition does require treatment, other options now exist that are less invasive than a hysterectomy, which is, after all, major surgery requiring several days in the hospital followed by about six weeks of recuperation at home. One such procedure is a myomectomy, in which the fibroids are surgically removed but the uterus is left intact. Different myomectomy procedures may be used, some more complex than others. Overall, however, a myomectomy is a more complicated surgical procedure than a hysterectomy. Any woman contemplating a myomectomy should select a surgeon who has performed many such operations and continues to do them regularly. She should also be aware of two major drawbacks of this procedure: The fibroids may return, which means additional surgery may be needed later on, and the

Healing the Pain

uterus may be damaged, making a subsequent pregnancy difficult or dangerous.

Natural health practitioners point out that fibroids may be related to lifestyle habits, such as a high-fat diet and too much stress, both of which can trigger high estrogen levels and stimulate fibroid growth. To stabilize estrogen production, these practitioners advise consuming a diet that is low in quantities of meat, dairy products, alcohol, and sugar, and practicing stress-relieving techniques such as relaxation, guided imagery, or meditation. Another alternative therapy for treating fibroids is Oriental medicine, which approaches treating the problem with a combination of acupuncture and herbal remedies in an effort to restore balanced body energy and sound health.

Fibromyalgia

Fibromyalgia is one of the more bewildering pain conditions. Many doctors know little about it; others choose to ignore it, believing it's not a real ailment. But the painful symptoms of fibromyalgia are profoundly real to the three to five million people in the United States (at least 80 percent of them women) who are compelled to live with them.

People with fibromyalgia feel as if they ache all over. The pain is centered in muscles and in the fibers that connect muscles to bones or other muscles. To diagnose the condition, a doctor will apply pressure to 18 points on the body. If at least 11 of these are painful, fibromyalgia is a possible diagnosis, according to guidelines established by the American College of

Rheumatology. (But a doctor won't necessarily rule out fibromyalgia if several points hurt, even if they are fewer than the standard of 11, and widespread pain exists elsewhere in the body.)

Fibromyalgia pain may be experienced as a burning, radiating, sore, stiff, aching, or gnawing sensation. The pain may range from mild to severe and may be found on both sides of the body as well as above and below the waist. To indicate a diagnosis of fibromyalgia, the pain must persist for at least three months.

In addition to the "aching all over" sensation, another key symptom is difficulty in sleeping. More than 90 percent of people with fibromyalgia suffer from fatigue. They sleep poorly at night, or even if they do get a good night's sleep, they awaken feeling tired. Other common symptoms might include:

- Depression or anxiety
- Headaches, including tension headaches and migraines
- Irritable bladder
- Irritable bowel syndrome
- Premenstrual tensions
- Mood changes
- Difficulty concentrating
- Numbness or tingling
- Sensitivity to cold
- A sensation of swelling or bloating, despite the absence of actual physical swelling
- Temporomandibular disorder

Because of the pervasive pain throughout the body, many people confuse fibromyalgia with some form of arthritis. But fibromyalgia, unlike arthritis, is not a disease of the joints.

Although fibromyalgia is not life-threatening, it can seriously impair a person's ability to work or engage in other normal daily activities. Relationships may be strained, as it's difficult for family members and friends to understand what is happening. Indeed, that may be one of the most difficult aspects of the disease: Others have a hard time believing that something is genuinely wrong because the person with fibromyalgia appears fine and healthy.

What to Do for Fibromyalgia

The cause of fibromyalgia has not been discovered, nor has a cure for it been found. And fibromyalgia does not go away. But someone living with this chronic pain condition can learn ways to cope with it.

One of the first steps, and for many people the most frustrating, is learning to adapt to chronic pain. That's especially tough for people who are used to leading a highly active life. With fibromyalgia, you may need more time to do daily activities. Depending on the severity of your condition, the strenuous activities you enjoyed in the past, such as hiking or skiing, don't necessarily have to be abandoned. But you will need to pace yourself and be aware of signs of fatigue and excessive stress. And though you may have to cut some activities from your life, with planning and creativity you can still participate in many of the activities you enjoy.

Medical experts advise that exercise is a crucial part of therapy for fibromyalgia. A sedentary life will only make the pain worse in the long run. High-impact exercises such as jogging should be avoided. But walking, swimming, and other low-impact forms of exercise are excellent for keeping up strength and preventing pain from getting worse.

Doctors may prescribe a low dose of an antidepressant to relieve pain and help you sleep better. Over-the-counter pain medications, however, may not do much to help the chronic pain of fibromyalgia, giving little and temporary relief. And long-term use of such medication may induce serious side effects. (See the chapter on over-the-counter medications.)

Biofeedback, relaxation, imagery, hypnosis, and meditation can also be used to manage how you perceive and respond to the pain and daily limitations brought on by fibromyalgia.

Combining several approaches may increase the chances for success. For example, consider a referral from your doctor to a physical therapist who will develop an exercise program, help from a psychologist to learn relaxation techniques, and consul-tation with a doctor who is knowledgeable about treating chronic pain conditions. Pain clinics usually offer this team approach to a problem such as fibromyalgia.

Gout

Long described as the disease of kings, gout once was thought to be an affliction that plagued rich men who ate and drank too much. In fact, gout strikes people of both sexes, of all economic classes. The old stereotype, however, has a few grains of truth: Men older than age 40 account for about 90 percent of gout sufferers. And obesity and alcohol abuse are risk factors for gout, as is a diet rich in purines, a substance found in organ meats, sardines, anchovies, dried peas, and beans. In addition, occupational exposure to lead, certain drugs for high blood pressure, family history of gout, and trauma may boost the risk of this disease.

As a joint disease, gout is actually a form of arthritis. Usually it strikes in the joint of the big toe; it also appears in the heel, instep, or Achilles tendon. Sometimes, especially in the case of recurrent attacks, gout can show up in the elbow, fingers, internal organs, knee, pelvis, shoulder, spine, or wrist. The conditions that lead to gout may exist for years, but the first attack often strikes suddenly, seemingly out of nowhere.

The root of the problem is uric acid, which comes from the foods we eat and from our body's normal metabolism. All of us have uric acid in our system. But for some people, the body's metabolism of uric acid goes awry, resulting in excessive levels of this substance in the bloodstream. Some, but not all, people with high levels of uric acid ultimately get gout, which develops when the uric acid forms crystals that lodge in the joint. As irritation sets in, the skin over the joint becomes red and swollen, and gout pain hits. Fever may be an accompanying symptom.

The reason gout commonly strikes in the big toe and other foot areas, especially in the first attack, is that uric-acid crystals more easily form at lower temperatures. The body's extremities, such as the feet, tend to be cooler than other body parts. Walking and standing also put stress on our feet much of the time.

A gout attack may last days or weeks and then subside. But usually a second attack comes months or years later, bringing more pain than the time before and doing more damage to the joint. Over time, the attacks become more frequent. If the condition is left

Healing the Pain

untreated, uric-acid crystals eventually may form tophi (gritty, chalky deposits) that can result in serious damage to joints, kidneys, or other organs.

What to Do for Gout Pain

First, a doctor should make sure that gout is really the problem. To rule out other conditions with goutlike symptoms, the doctor can extract a small amount of fluid from the big toe or other affected joint and test for uric-acid crystals. Once the diagnosis is certain, treatment can begin.

There is no cure for gout, but it can be kept under control. When an attack hits, nonsteroidal anti-inflammatory drugs (NSAIDs) can reduce pain and swelling. Two NSAIDs commonly used by doctors are indomethacin and naproxen. Another medication, given by injection, is ACTH (adrenocorticotrophic hormone). If none of these drugs work to ease the pain, the doctor may advise using steroids. To prevent future attacks, the doctor may prescribe various medications that control uric-acid levels.

A commonly used herbal medicine for the pain of gout is a combination of garlic and devil's claw.

Because cold/heat therapy eases the pain of other forms of arthritis, many people assume the same would be true for gout. But, in fact, cold and heat can make gout worse. Heat increases circulation and thus may worsen the irritation brought on by the uric-acid crystals. Cold may cause the formation of more crystals.

To reduce your risk of gout, lose any excess weight. Studies show that for a man between ages 25 and 35, ten extra pounds doubles his risk. Ten more pounds doubles his risk again, and so on. (No studies have been done for women.) Drinking too much alcohol also boosts the risk of gout. But drinking plenty of water (six to eight glasses a day) offers some protection by diluting uric acid and helping the kidneys remove it.

Other research studies have linked gout to diabetes and high blood pressure. This reemphasizes the point made earlier: If you have an attack of what you think may be gout, see your doctor to verify the condition—and to spot other, potentially life-threatening health conditions that may have triggered the gout attack.

Headache

Nearly everyone gets a headache now and then. But for some peo-ple, due to frequency, intensity, or both, headaches constitute a health problem. According to the National Headache Foundation in Chicago, about 45 million Americans suffer from recurring headaches—defined as headaches that strike at least once a month. Whether we suffer headaches occasionally or regularly, most of us try to carry on with our daily lives—even if functioning below par. For the roughly 17 million Americans prone to migraine attacks, however, the pain can be incapacitating. In some cases, migraine sufferers must limit activity to no more than living quietly in a dimly lit room, perhaps for as long as several days.

While there are several types of headaches, here we will focus on three of the more common ones: tension headaches, migraines, and cluster headaches.

Tension headaches

Accounting for roughly 90 percent of all headaches, this is the type most of us know first hand. A tension headache is felt as a dull, nonthrobbing pain in the forehead and temples, at the back of the head, or encircling the head in a band. Muscles of the neck and jaw may also feel tight, even knotted. The headache comes on due to tension in the face, jaw, and neck muscles, which in turn may be caused by factors such as stress, poor posture, lack of sleep, and poor diet.

Some researchers prefer to use the term "tension-type headache," indicating their doubts about whether muscle tension is truly the root cause. Perhaps other factors, such as brain chemicals, may play a part in triggering this type of headache. Research continues in this area; in the meantime, the old term "tension headache" remains in widespread use.

Migraines

Migraine pain is throbbing, usually located on one side of the head, and ranges from mild to severe. Icy hands, nausea, pallor, sensitivity to light or sound, sweating, or vomiting can be accompanying symptoms. The pain can last for a matter of minutes or as long as several days and can be severe enough to force the migraine sufferer to put his or her life activities on hold until the attack passes.

About 10 percent of those afflicted with migraines experience auras before the attack, thus providing them with a warning signal. An aura may take forms such as having blurry vision, seeing flashing lights, feeling sensations of tingling or numbness, hearing noises, or smelling odors.

Healing the Pain

Some experts feel that a migraine is a vascular headache, meaning it involves changes in blood vessels in the head. Various theories exist as to why these changes occur, though the tendency toward migraines seems to be inherited. While migraines are more common in boys than girls in the younger years, in adulthood women are three times as likely to get migraines as men. Migraine triggers include food allergies, food additives, stress, hormonal shifts, smoking, and disrupted eating or sleeping routines.

Cluster headaches

Less common than migraines but sometimes more severe, cluster headaches manifest themselves as a steady, burning, and penetrating pain on one side of the head. They are often centered around the eye and sometimes the forehead, temple, cheek, jaw, teeth, neck, or ear.

Sufferers commonly describe the experience as "like a knife in the eye." Cluster headaches get their name from the fact that they occur in groups of as many as six a day, possibly more, lasting for weeks or months. Other symptoms include sweating in the face, a runny nose on the same side of the head as the pain, and tearing of the eye. The pain erupts suddenly, often two or three hours after falling asleep, and can last up to a couple of hours.

The exact causes of cluster headaches are unknown, but they are five times more common among men than women. People who smoke or drink heavily are also more apt to get them.

What to Do for Headache Pain

Several different headache therapies are available, depending on your health care preferences, what type of headache you're treating, and what works best for you. Some people find headache relief with behavioral/psychological techniques such as biofeedback, relaxation, imagery, hypnosis, or meditation. But the first step is to see your doctor for a professional evaluation.

Biofeedback involves being connected by means of electrodes attached to the surface of your skin to an instrument that provides cues, or feedback, about what's happening in your body. By learning relaxation or imagery in conjunction with biofeedback techniques, you can develop the ability to control certain body functions. For example, to ward off a tension headache, you might use biofeedback to relax your head and neck muscles. Stretching the neck and shoulder area tends to ease the discomfort. Hypnosis has also been used with success in learning how to relax and how to control pain through mental capacities not normally available to us. Yet another technique is meditation, a mental-focusing exercise through which we can gain the ability to control stresses and tensions that can trigger headaches or migraines.

For those who prefer to seek relief through medication, over-the-counter medications such as aspirin and other NSAIDs (non-steroidal anti-inflammatory drugs) can be extremely useful for treating headaches and migraines. More severe headaches may require prescription painkillers. A popular new drug for migraines is sumatriptan, which once was available only by injection, but is now available in an easier-to-take tablet form. It should not, however, be used by people with heart

Healing the Pain

disease or high blood pressure. Another medication available in a nasal spray, called dihydroergotamine mesylate (DHE), is expected to be available soon for general use. It shows promise of being as effective as sumatriptan but with fewer side effects, though it's not advised for regular use by people with diabetes or poor circulation. The search for an "ideal" migraine medication continues.

If you get chronic headaches, you may benefit from keeping a headache diary. It could be a simple notebook in which you record lifestyle habits and headache history. Rate the intensity of your headaches from one to three for mild, moderate, and severe. Then write down what you ate, when you went to bed, what sorts of stress you experienced, what medications you took, and so on. Over time, you may begin to notice pat-

terns linked to your headaches that may lead to some relief. It is also important to check with a physician to be certain that your headache is not the result of a serious condition.

Herpes (Genital)

Since the 1960s, the incidence of genital herpes has soared in the United States. An estimated 31 million people were infected as of 1991, according to the Centers for Disease Control and Prevention. And as many as half a million new cases are reported each year.

Genital herpes is a viral infection caused by herpes simplex virus type II. That's a relative of herpes simplex type I, which is the cause of cold sores on the mouth, face, and lips. The type II herpes shows up as sores in or on the penis,

Healing the Pain

vagina, cervix, thighs, and sometimes the buttocks. The infection starts as itching, burning, or tingling in the genital area, followed by painful blisters that erupt after a few days to form ulcers, also painful, that persist for one to three weeks. These sores may make urination irritating and difficult. Other symptoms might include swollen lymph glands in the groin area, fever, and an all-around feeling of being ill.

Transmission of herpes from one person to another occurs through contact, such as oral or genital sex. The infected person passes the virus to another during its active stage, when sores are present, or during the preactive stage, which is characterized by itching and irritation. But transmission might also occur even before the infected person is experiencing any of the preactive symptoms. The partner

of the infected person is likely to have a herpes outbreak within a couple of days to two weeks of sexual contact.

The most troubling aspect of herpes is that once it's in your system, it's there to stay. It has inactive, or dormant, periods during which you're symptom free, but new episodes can erupt at any time. Usually the first episode is the most painful.

Herpes can lead to other serious complications as well. For example, women with herpes may be at greater than normal risk for cervical cancer. Thus, any woman with herpes should be diligent about having an annual Pap smear and pelvic examination. And all women of child-bearing age should be aware that a newborn baby can get herpes from an infected mother during birth.

What triggers reactivation of dormant herpes? Doctors believe various factors may play a role. You might be more vulnerable to recurrences after a serious illness—when resistance is down. Emotional stress can weaken your immune system's ability to suppress growth of the virus. People on immunosuppressive or anticancer drugs also are more susceptible to recurrences. Menstruation, sunbathing, and genital trauma can also trigger recurrences.

If you suspect you might have herpes, see your doctor for an accurate diagnosis and to rule out the presence of other sexually transmitted diseases.

What to Do for Genital Herpes

There is no cure for herpes, but you can take steps to relieve your discomfort during the virus' active periods and reduce the likelihood of recurrences.

A doctor's first line of treatment will be an antiviral prescription medication such as acyclovir, which is taken orally. Doctors agree on the effectiveness of this medication for treating first episodes, but opinions differ as to its usefulness for recurrences. Some doctors recommend long-term use of these antiviral agents as a preventive measure in the case of frequent recurrences. Even so, most experts advise interrupting the medication every one to three years to verify that its continued use is justified.

In addition, taking an over-the-counter pain medication can help relieve your painful symptoms. Another way to soothe discomfort is to take a warm bath with a tablespoon of salt added to the bath water.

To prevent irritating the herpes sores, wear cotton underwear, which doesn't trap heat and moisture in the genital area the way synthetic underwear does. Similarly, don't wear tight pants. After bathing, be sure you pat (don't rub) your genitals thoroughly dry. Use a separate towel to dry your genitals to lessen the risk of spreading the virus to other parts of the body, such as your mouth or eyes. And don't share towels with anyone during active herpes periods.

Avoid sex (oral or genital) during active or preactive phases. That means no sex, not even with a condom: A condom might or might not prevent herpes from spreading from an infected man to his partner; it does not stop the spread from an infected woman to her partner. During inactive periods, you can resume normal sex-ual relations—but be sure to always use a condom and inform your partner.

To reduce the likelihood of recurrences, keep yourself in good overall health. Maintaining a diary of lifestyle habits might help to determine the substances or conditions that trigger herpes recurrences for you. Eat a good diet, get enough sleep, keep stress and tension under control, exercise regularly, don't smoke, and don't use drugs or alcohol. Meditation, imagery, and relaxation techniques can help you cope with stress. Acupuncture and herbs may help to suppress reactivation of herpes.

Menstrual Cramps

For many women, menstrual cramps are like the bills they get in the mail every month. Here they come, on schedule, whether or not you feel ready to deal with them. Medical experts don't know for sure what causes all menstrual cramps. But one common cause is uterine contractions induced by prostaglandins, a hormonelike body chemical. Prostaglandins reach peak levels in the uterus during menstruation. The contractions constrict uterine blood vessels, reducing the blood supply to the uterus and thus causing pain. Some women have mild cramps that allow them to go on with their activities as usual. At the other end of the spectrum are women whose menstrual cramps are so severe that they can do little else but take refuge in bed for a day or two every month. Along with the cramps, some women experience other symptoms of menstrual pain, among them backaches, breast tenderness, constipation, diarrhea, dizziness, fainting, fatigue, headaches, nausea, and vomiting.

In technical medical terms, menstrual pain can be categorized as either primary or secondary dysmenorrhea. The former is the more common, once-a-month variety (as described above), while the latter is usually due to some other health problem such as uterine fibroids, endometriosis, pelvic inflammatory disease (see other sections in this book for more information on these conditions), a congenital abnormality in the uterus, or pain caused by an intrauterine device (IUD) for birth control. Symptoms of secondary dysmenorrhea can include feelings of pressure or pain in the pelvic area or the back, fever, heavy clots, heavy menstrual bleeding, and irregular menstruation. If you have been menstruating for years and these symptoms appear suddenly, you might suspect secondary dysmenorrhea, with one of the underlying causes mentioned above. Don't try to self-treat any of these conditions. Your symptoms warrant a visit to your health care practitioner for an examination and diagnosis.

Not only do the cramps experienced by one woman differ in severity from those of another, but the nature of cramps can change during the course of one individual's lifetime. For instance, some women find that their cramps gradually get less painful as they age, while for others the opposite is true.

Sometimes women get cramps at the midpoint of their menstrual cycle. In such cases, pain is triggered by ovulation, which occurs when the egg follicle ruptures and releases the egg. Mild pain and even a little bleeding can accompany ovulation.

What to Do for Menstrual Cramps

If your doctor concludes that your menstrual cramps are not due to any underlying health problem, you can safely treat them yourself with simple at-home therapies. For example, you can apply a heating pad or hot water bottle to your back or abdomen. Or you could sit in a warm bath. Some women find applying cold provides more relief, while others are helped by alternating cool and warm sitz baths. (To take a sitz bath, sit in a tub filled with just four or five inches of water.)

More than a few women turn to herbs for the relief of cramps. One suggestion from herbalists is a ginger tea made with a teaspoon of freshly grated ginger root simmered in a cup of hot water. Chamomile is reported to have value as a cramp-reliever, either in a tea or as an oil massaged into the lower abdomen. Lavender oil is also said to be helpful when rubbed into the area of the lower abdomen. If your cramps are more severe, try valerian in capsule or as a tincture.

Lifestyle habits can help to reduce both your susceptibility to menstrual cramps and their severity. Note, however, that to get real benefits these should be ongoing habits, not just measures to try to "clean up your act" during your period. Eat a healthy diet that is low in fat, sugar, alcohol, and caffeine (which is found not just in coffee, but in some teas, cola drinks, and chocolate). Be sure to include plenty of whole grains in your diet and a generous supply of fruits and vegetables. Adequate levels of calcium and magnesium also help to ward off cramps.

Get regular exercise all month long; that includes during your period. Exercise during your period can trigger the release of brain chemicals called endorphins which are natural mood-elevators and pain-killers. But there is no need to overdo it: A brisk walk, jog, swim, or bicycle ride can be enough.

If you smoke, menstrual cramps provide one more reason to quit. A study published in *Epidemiology* in 1994 found that women who smoked 10 to 30 cigarettes a day were at double the risk for cramps as women who didn't smoke. Women who smoked for 10 to 20 years tripled their risk of cramps.

Controlling stress is also a factor. Relaxation techniques, imagery, and meditation can boost your ability to cope with stress. Some women like the combination of relaxation and exercise they get with such practices as yoga or *Tai Chi Chuan*.

NSAIDs (nonsteroidal anti-inflammatory drugs) such as aspirin and ibuprofen are the most commonly used home remedy for the relief of menstrual cramps. They inhibit the prostaglandin-induced changes in the uterus. (See the chapter on over-the-counter medications.)

Muscle Cramps

Muscle cramps don't lead to permanent disability or damage, but they can be bothersome and painful nonetheless. And they can be a bit baffling. Sometimes you have a good idea what you did to set off a cramp—overdoing a jogging session, for example, or playing an overzealous game of volleyball. At other times, muscle cramps, or spasms, seem to hit for no apparent reason. A cramping muscle can even jolt you out of a sound sleep in the middle of the night.

But as much as it may seem so at times, muscle cramps aren't just a matter of your body playing tricks on you. Day in and day out our muscles expand and contract repeatedly as we go through our daily motions. When we want a muscle to contract, the brain sends a message via the nerves to that muscle. In and around the muscle are minerals—including sodium, calcium, and potassium—that pass the brain's message along the muscle. Proper muscle contraction and relaxation depend on a sufficient supply of minerals, as well as fat, sugar, and oxygen.

Sometimes this process doesn't work quite the way it should. As a result, the muscle goes into a spasm, or cramp, which interferes with blood flow to the muscle and causes pain. The pain may cause more spasms, further inhibiting blood flow to the muscle and causing even more pain. The muscle then becomes stuck in the contracting phase of the contraction-relaxation cycle.

Some of the most common locations for cramps include the legs, ankles, neck, back, fingers, toes, and along the side of the torso just below the rib cage (commonly called a side stitch). Several factors that can lead to muscle cramps include:

Overuse of the muscle. This could result from an excessive burst of activity or from movement that's not particularly strenuous but that uses the same muscle over and over again for a period of time. The cramp might pop up right away, in an hour or two, or even a day or more later, triggered by some minor exertion of an already overused muscle. For instance, you might feel fine after playing hard in your Saturday softball game, but on Monday you're hit with a leg cramp while running up a flight of stairs. Or a cramp can come on when you do nothing more strenuous than turn over in your sleep.

Dehydration. Fluids are essential for your body's muscles to contract and relax normally anytime, especially during hot weather. Even if you don't feel thirsty, you may be short of fluids needed for healthy muscle functioning.

Certain medications. Some medications deplete the body's supply of potassium, thus affecting the contraction-relaxation process. Among such medications are diuretics (taken to lower blood pressure) and corticosteroids.

Tight clothing. Pants, belts, shoes, and other items of clothing that are too tight can interfere with normal blood flow to the muscles, which can spur cramps.

Calcium shortage. An inadequate intake of calcium has been linked to muscle cramps, especially ones that occur at night.

What to Do for Muscle Cramps

When a cramp hits, you hardly need urging to stop what you're doing. The instinct to stop is an important one because you can injure the muscle if you attempt to keep going in an effort to work out the cramp.

The next step is to *gently* stretch and massage the cramped muscle. You want to stretch it in the opposite direction from the way it's contracted. Emphasis here is on the word *gently*. If you overdo the stretch, you could injure the muscle. Massage can loosen up the tight muscle and enhance the

blood flow to it, but massaging with too much pressure could inhibit blood flow, rather than increase it. Once the cramp has loosened its grip, don't dive right back into the activity you were doing. Walk around for a while to get the blood flowing to the affected muscle.

Here are a few examples of stretches intended to ease specific types of muscle cramps:

Calves. Place your palms against a wall, at shoulder level, while you stand with your good leg about a foot from the wall and your cramped leg about six inches farther away from the wall. Keep your feet flat on the floor while you lean toward the wall. Bend the good leg and keep the cramped leg straight. Hold for half a minute. Don't bounce. Repeat a few times until the cramp loosens.

Toes (curled under). If your toes are cramped in a curled-under position, sit down on a mat or the floor and place the affected foot on the knee of the other leg. Grab the cramped toes (use your right hand for your right foot) so that your fingers are over the toes and your thumb is underneath them. Use your thumb to rub the toes from the ball of the foot to the toes. Then move your hand so you can stretch the toes toward your ankle with your fingers (in other words, the toes will be stretched toward the top side of your foot).

Toes (straightened). Position yourself as described above. This time simply bend the toes downward so they are in more of a curled position.

Hamstrings (muscles on the rear side of the thigh). Lie down on your back on the floor. Let your uncramped leg remain straight on the floor while you grasp the cramped leg by the knee and pull it toward your chest.

Better than coping with muscle cramps once they grab hold is doing all you can to prevent them. One major step in that direction is performing regular stretching exercises to lengthen your muscles. This helps keep the muscles loose and therefore less likely to cramp. The best times to stretch are before and after exercise as well as at bedtime. And don't forget to warm up your muscles before stretching, which you can do by taking a warm bath or a short walk.

You can also help to elude cramps by getting enough water, which means at least six to eight 8-ounce glasses a day. You need more—perhaps twice as much—when it's very hot or you're exercising.

Healing the Pain

Nerve (Injury) Pain

Nerve injuries have many causes, ranging from a disease, such as diabetes, to a major trauma, such as a gunshot wound. *Neuralgia*, or neuropathic pain, is the medical term for pain due to an injured or damaged nerve. Just as there are many different nerves in the body, there are many forms of neuralgia. Characteristics and severity of neuralgic pain vary widely. Here we will look at some representative examples of this disorder.

Peripheral Neuropathy

This is an impairment of the peripheral nerves, the nerves other than those of the brain and spinal cord. Peripheral neuropathy may be due to a multitude of causes, among them alcoholism, anemia, diabetes mellitus, overexposure to industrial or farm chemicals, or certain vitamin deficiencies.

Diabetic neuropathy, for instance, often first appears in the feet. As in other neuropathies, it can be felt as a tingling sensation that evolves into numbness and pain. The feeling, described as burning, is made worse by activity such as walking. Numbness may sound harmless, but in fact it carries a substantial risk because a person may develop a problem and not realize it. Without knowing anything is wrong, he or she may develop skin ulcers on the feet that become infected. These ulcers may be triggered by excessive pressure on a certain part of the foot, a puncture wound, or a foreign object lodged in the shoe, unnoticed by its wearer. Severe cases of diabetic neuropathy can lead to amputation, particularly when accompanied by poor circulation.

Another outcome can be severe foot deformities, which might result not only from ulcers on pressure points, but also from severe foot fractures or dislocations. Again, the lack of feeling is the culprit, because people with diabetes may unknowingly traumatize their feet, resulting in injury.

Trigeminal Neuralgia

Trigeminal neuralgia affects the trigeminal nerve, a major nerve in the face that controls sensation to the teeth, mouth, face, and nasal cavity, as well as movement of the jaw. When trigeminal neuralgia (also called tic douloureux) strikes, the victim may assume he or she has a crushing toothache. Studies show that people often seek—and receive—dental treatment, even root canal procedures, before discovering that the problem isn't with their teeth after all.

Words such as *stabbing* or *jabbing* are often used to describe the pain, which affects areas on the face or in the mouth and can vary from mild to excruciating. While pain attacks can be intense, usually the pain goes into remission for months, even years. In many cases, however, episodes become more frequent over time. And the pain can be serious enough to interfere with normal activities, such as talking, eating, or brushing the teeth.

Trigeminal neuralgia most commonly strikes older people (it is most frequently seen in those over age 70). Though the exact cause is unknown, a contributing factor may be a blood vessel that puts pressure on the trigeminal nerve. Sometimes other health disorders, such as multiple sclerosis or a tumor, can also trigger trigeminal neuralgia.

Postherpetic Neuralgia

Long after an outbreak of shingles is over, pain can linger in the form of postherpetic neuralgia. Shingles is caused by a virus, the herpes zoster virus (the same one responsible for chicken pox), that appears as a rash that erupts into blisters on the skin along the course of an affected nerve. In some cases, especially in people over age 60, the nerve endings inflamed by the shingles virus trigger postherpetic neuralgia, a chronic and severe pain that can last for more than a year. (See the section on shingles for more information.)

What to Do for Nerve-Injury Pain

Treatments for nerve injuries vary as much as the injuries themselves. The location of the damaged nerve, the severity of pain, and the underlying factors causing the nerve disorder all have an impact on the type of treatment to be used.

Diabetic Neuropathy

For diabetic neuropathy, the best strategy is prevention. That means diligent foot care. Anyone with diabetes needs to be particularly conscientious about checking the feet daily, looking for sores, blisters, cuts, and so on. Washing your feet every day is also critical in keeping them free of problems. And you should apply a cream afterward to prevent the skin from cracking. Whenever you notice a sore that's not healing properly, see your doctor immediately.

To protect your feet, avoid walking around without shoes. And when it comes to buying shoes, be sure to choose a pair that fits well and provides ample cushioning. Because shoes lose much of their cushioning capacity after you've walked in them for a few hours, changing shoes once or twice each day will also help.

If you develop diabetic neuropathy, you may find relief from the pain by applying a cream containing capsaicin, the chemical that gives chili peppers their heat. A study reported in *Archives of Internal Medicine* in 1991 involved 252 patients and found that, compared with an inactive cream, capsaicin cream applied four times a day resulted in a statistically significant improvement in pain relief along with a decrease in pain intensity. The only side effects were temporary burning at the application site and some sneezing and coughing.

Transcutaneous electrical stimulation, or TENS, is another pain therapy that can be helpful for relieving peripheral nerve pain, including that of diabetic neuropathy. In TENS, electrodes placed on the skin send a low-intensity current to targeted nerves underneath the skin.

Trigeminal Neuralgia

Doctors rely on the prescription medications baclofen (Lioresal) and carbamazepine (Tegretol) as major treatments for trigeminal neuralgia. But if drug therapy doesn't do the job for you, surgery may be advised. Recent studies show good success rates with microvascular decompression, a surgical procedure that involves separating or removing the blood vessel that's pressing on the trigeminal root.

Among alternative therapies, acupuncture reportedly can be effective with trigeminal neuralgia. Inserting fine needles at acupoints is designed to stimulate the flow of life energy and lead to pain relief.

Postherpetic Neuralgia

Treatments can range from cold/heat therapies to nerve blocks, depending on the severity

inserted under anesthesia through a tiny incision in the abdomen, to get a better view of the cyst. Laparoscopy, as the procedure is called, can also guide the doctor in performing a biopsy, which involves removing a small amount of tissue from the cyst for testing. Such methods will help diagnose malignancy. If malignancy is found, surgery would be performed, perhaps involving removal of the uterus as well as the ovaries.

In certain instances, doctors will take a more aggressive diagnostic approach right from the start, foregoing the wait-and-see period. This might occur if a cyst is larger than four inches in diameter or if it develops after menopause. In the case of a younger woman with a twisted ovary and cyst who is experiencing extreme pain, surgery should be undertaken as soon as possible. Even

though this kind of surgery is not often successful, it is important to try to save the ovary and preserve the woman's capacity to bear children. Surgery is also desirable to prevent damage from dead or dying tissue, which may lead to inflammation and infection.

Some women are prone to recurrent ovarian cysts, which can be a sign that some lifestyle changes are needed, such as reducing stress and improving your diet. Oriental medicine, including acupuncture and herbal remedies, has been reported to help restore balance in the body and, therefore, halt recurrent cysts.

Pelvic Inflammatory Disease

Health statistics indicate that approximately one million women in the United States contract pelvic inflammatory disease (PID) each year. Experts claim that many more women have the disease but are not even aware of it. This is either because they are symptom-free and don't realize anything is wrong or because their doctors aren't familiar with PID and miss the diagnosis. Still, PID can lead to serious complications, even death.

PID is an infection that usually affects the uterus, the fallopian tubes, the ovaries, or some combination of the three. The most common site of infection is the fallopian tubes. If left untreated, PID can result in blockage and scarring of the fallopian tubes. This closes off the passageway for the egg or sperm, which in turn prevents fertilization and precludes pregnancy.

Blockage of the fallopian tube can become life-threatening when a fertilized egg becomes trapped in the tube and starts to grow. (This is called an ectopic pregnancy, or a pregnancy outside the uterus.) If the fertilized egg keeps growing, the tube may burst, an emergency that can be fatal if surgery isn't performed immediately. Any woman who has had PID in the past and becomes pregnant should inform her doctor, who will check to be sure an ectopic pregnancy hasn't developed.

Of women who have one episode of PID, roughly 12 percent end up infertile; among those who have three or more episodes, the infertility rate is more than 50 percent.

The two most common causes of PID are two sexually transmitted diseases (STDs): chlamydia and gonorrhea. Chlamydia has become a common STD, with about 4 million new cases reported each year. Often a woman with chlamydia has no symptoms and isn't aware that she has the disease. But if it's not treated, the infection can move to the upper reproductive tract, resulting in PID. A recent study reported in *The New England Journal of Medicine* in 1996 found that the incidence of PID could be cut by more than half if sexually active women were routinely screened for chlamydia during their annual pelvic examinations. In PID due to chlamydia, a woman's symptoms may be mild, at most. She may have no pain, or only mild pain in the pelvic area, in the lower back, or only during sexual intercourse. Vaginal discharge may be thicker or thinner than usual. PID due to chlamydia can lead to severe damage, however, even though the noticeable symptoms are mild or nonexistent.

Gonorrhea-caused PID has more blatant symptoms, including chills, fever, severe pelvic pain, vaginal bleeding, and a puslike vaginal discharge.

Symptoms depend not only on the type of microorganism, but also on where the infection is, how long you've had it, and your general state of health. The wide variability of symptoms, or lack of them, can make it tough to diagnose PID. Some doctors, unfortunately, write off chronic, mild pelvic pain as just one of those "woman's problems" that's of no real consequence. If you believe this is happening to you, complain to your doctor. If that doesn't help, find another doctor. To aid in the diagnosis of PID, a physician can take a blood test and a culture of cells from the cervix for laboratory testing.

What to Do for PID

Getting rid of PID requires 10 to 14 days of antibiotics, which must be taken for the full time period even if symptoms disappear. Your male sexual partner must also be treated; otherwise you and your partner could repeatedly reinfect each other. Sometimes antibiotics can trigger a vaginal yeast infection. Acidophilus, taken in the form of yogurt or a supplement, may lessen the likelihood of that occurring.

Sometimes PID treatment requires hospitalization. If the infection has not responded to antibiotics, or if it's widespread, you can receive intravenous doses of antibiotics, which more efficiently work their way to the site of infection. If this method fails to bring results, your doctor may wish to do a laparoscopy. This involves the insertion of a small tube through an incision in the abdomen. Guided by a viewing device called a laparoscope, a doctor can drain an abscess, cut away scar tissue, or extract a fluid sample for laboratory testing.

A hot bath or hot pad applied to your lower abdomen can ease pain and help stimulate blood flow to the area, which aids healing. Raspberry leaf tea is an herbal remedy said to strengthen the reproductive system. Eating well, getting plenty of rest, and reducing stress can also assist the healing process. Be aware, however, that these measures are intended only to make you more comfortable while you are eradicating the infection. They are not cures for PID, which is a serious infection that can have severe complications.

To prevent PID, be sure your male partner uses a condom. And use birth control other than an IUD (intrauterine device), which has been linked to greater risk for PID.

Postsurgical Pain

For someone facing an operation, one of the major concerns is coping with the pain that often follows surgery. The types of pains and discomforts you experience depend on such factors as the type of surgery, the anesthetic used during the operation, and your general state of health.

Besides the pain at the incision site itself, you may feel various discomforts in the aftermath of the anesthesia. Different people have different reactions, but some of the adverse effects might include dizziness, nausea, restlessness, disorientation, numbness, ringing in the ears, and slurred speech.

Before surgery, talk to your doctor so you know what to expect. What sort of pain might you have? How long might it last? What anesthetics will be used before and during the operation? What are the possible lingering effects of these? What pain medications will be used after surgery? How long will they be needed, and what side effects can be expected?

Be sure you fully understand the answers to these questions and the reasons behind the surgeon's decisions before the surgery is performed. The last thing you need when you're recuperating is anxiety about any of these issues.

When you're in the recovery stage, be straightforward with your doctor about the pain you're feeling. All too often, patients feel reluctant to talk about their pain, fearing they'll come across as a whiner or a wimp. But look at it this way: You have a perfect right to expect adequate pain management after surgery. (See the section on surgery for more information). For the doctor to do his or her best to make you comfortable, you have to describe your pain as clearly and accurately as you can.

What to Do for Postsurgical Pain

Pain management may be required while you're in the hospital and for some time thereafter. For milder postoperative pain, ordinary over-the-counter painkillers may be sufficient. For more severe postoperative pain, some hospitals offer special treatment. Ask your surgeon about the availability of such services at your hospital.

You might consider other therapies to use in conjunction with pain medications, or even to reduce your need for them. For instance, hypnosis has been found to be effective in controlling post

surgical pain and also aids healing. A study at Columbia University, reported in a 1995 issue of the *Journal of Alternative and Complementary Medicine*, found that self-hypnosis (used in combination with imagery, relaxation, and positive-thinking techniques) helped patients feel less tired and less depressed in the days following their coronary artery bypass operations. These patients underwent the therapy combination the night before surgery to enhance their ability to cope physically and psychologically with their postsurgical discomforts. Again, be sure to check into the availability of this approach well in advance of your surgery.

For some patients, transcutaneous electrical nerve stimulation (TENS) may help ease pain after surgery. (See the chapter on TENS for more information.)

Oriental medicine, using acupuncture and herbs, has been reported to offer relief for postoperative pain. Herbal practitioners recommend a combination of equal parts of tinctures of Siberian ginseng, ginkgo, milk thistle, and hawthorn to bolster the body's natural healing capabilities. Calendula oil or cream, applied to the skin, can enhance wound healing. However, be sure to discuss these remedies with your surgeon and get his or her approval before using any of these techniques.

Shingles

At a time when a childhood bout of chicken pox is only a distant memory, the disease can make a return visit that is even less welcome than your first encounter. This time the virus is in the form of an uncomfortable illness known as shingles.

Both chicken pox and shingles trace their cause to the varicella-zoster virus, one of the herpes family of viruses. After chicken pox strikes in childhood, the virus hibernates in nerve cells in your body. For one reason or another, the virus gets revived out of dormancy in some people, showing up decades later as shingles. Roughly 20 percent of those who had chicken pox as children end up with shingles, which usually appears after the age of 50.

The first noticeable symptom of shingles is usually pain at the site of the affected nerve. Or there may be a prickly, burning sensation in the skin over the nerve. Some people get other symptoms early on, such as headaches, stomach upset, chills, or a feeling of sluggishness. Others get none of these early signs, but first notice a reddish, itchy, blistery skin rash. Normally the rash appears in bands or strips on the skin. In fact, another name for shingles is herpes zoster, zoster being a Latin word meaning belt or girdle. The rash is often on just one side of the body, following the course of the affected nerve under the skin. Common locations include the rib area, neck, arms, or legs. Sometimes the rash appears on one side of the face, close to the eye, which can also become affected by the virus. This condition, known as ophthalmic zoster, can result in impaired vision if not treated quickly.

Why does the chicken-pox virus come back to haunt some people and not others? Medical experts don't know for sure what reactivates it. But possible triggers include a worn-down immune system, emotional stress, illness, injury, or the stress of major surgery. People with immune-system diseases such as AIDS are highly susceptible. Chemotherapy also affects the immune system and can sometimes set off a bout of shingles.

Usually shingles will run its course within a week or two. The blisters crust over, and the pain goes away. But in some cases, the pain lingers on in the form of a more serious disorder called postherpetic neuralgia (PHN). Estimates vary on how often this happens, but experts agree that it's more likely to occur if you are older when you contract shingles. For people who get shingles after age 50, for example, as many as half may end up with PHN.

The pain of PHN may be more severe than shingles and, unlike shingles, it can last for weeks or months. In some cases, especially when older people are affected, it can go on for years. People with

Healing the Pain

PHN may have skin so sensitive that even a light touch, such as contact with clothing or a change of temperature, can trigger extreme pain. The pain may come on as a sharp, stabbing pain. In other cases, PHN pain takes the form of a deep achy feeling that never lets up.

No matter what form it takes, the chronic pain is very difficult to bear, and a person may become prone to depression. In particularly difficult cases, suicide may be contemplated. Indeed, doctors say PHN is a major cause of pain-related suicide in the elderly, second in frequency only to suicide brought on by cancer pain.

Some people are concerned about catching shingles from someone else. But in order for that to happen, you would have to have direct contact with the fluid from the blistery sores. Thus, provided the sores are covered, the likelihood of the disease spreading is minimal. And even that limited risk lasts only until the blisters heal. Note, however, that someone who has never had chicken pox can catch that disease from someone who is infected with shingles.

What to Do for Shingles

The key point medical experts make about dealing with shingles is that the sooner treatment starts, the better. The first line of treatment is the use of one of several antiviral medications, which reduces pain, speeds healing, and fights the virus. These prescription medications are most effective if treatment begins within 48 hours of the outbreak of the rash.

Keeping the affected skin clean and dry is extremely important to avoid the risk of infection. To help relieve the pain, some doctors recommend a compress soaked with

Burow's solution. Apply it to the affected area for 15 minutes, then repeat the process four times a day.

As for shingles prevention, the best things you can do are to exercise and to eat a nutritious, balanced diet—two measures that help to keep your immunity strong and thus make you less prone to illness in general, shingles included.

PHN is more difficult to treat than shingles. Some doctors believe that use of the antiviral medications helps to reduce the chances that shingles will develop into PHN. But this is widely debated in the medical community. Another treatment thought to be effective for PHN is the injection of local anesthetic and steroid on the nerve during the acute stage of an attack.

Applying a cream containing capsaicin, the substance that gives chili peppers their heat, works in some people to relieve PHN pain. (Note: Capsaicin cream should not be used on open shingles sores, as the burning sensation of the medication itself can cause more pain.) The Burow's compress mentioned above also may help, as may calamine lotion. Both of these preparations are available over the counter.

Transcutaneous electrical nerve stimulation (TENS) is another therapy that's been helpful for some people suffering from PHN pain. TENS uses mild electrical impulses sent through electrodes placed on the skin. It's thought that these impulses either block pain signals from reaching the brain or stimulate the body's production of endorphins, its own natural painkilling chemicals.

Because PHN is difficult to treat, you may need to experiment with different therapies, or combinations of therapies, to find out what helps your individual situation. Not all treatments work for everyone. Remember, too, that the pain of PHN usually fades over time: For 70 to 80 percent of people with PHN, the pain vanishes within a year.

Shinsplints

Doctors and athletes alike use the term shinsplints to refer to just about any pain along the shinbone (or tibia) of the lower leg. At best, it's an imprecisely defined condition. One chief cause is muscle overuse. Running and jumping on hard surfaces—especially if you are out of training, have abruptly cranked up your workout to a more strenuous level, or wear worn-out athletic shoes—is another major risk factor for shinsplints. Joggers, aerobic dancers, football players, and gymnasts are just some of the athletes susceptible to this kind of injury.

Some sports-medicine specialists believe that the way your foot hits the ground when you're running has a great deal to do with developing shinsplints. As you run and jump, the arch of your foot rises and collapses in repeated cycles. It collapses to absorb the shock of your foot hitting the ground, and then as you roll up on your toes for the next step, the arch comes up to prepare for the next impact with the ground. If, on impact, your foot rolls too much to the inside, however, the arch's collapse-rise cycle doesn't work as it should. That puts undue stress on the muscle that attaches your arch to your shin bone. A small part tears loose from the bone, causing you to feel pain.

Usually shinsplints goes away within a couple of weeks. But at

Healing the Pain

times it can linger and be tough to shake.

Shinsplints can be mistaken for the more serious injuries of stress fracture and compartment syndrome. A stress fracture is a microscopic crack in the shinbone that can be so small it can't be seen on an X ray, though it will reveal itself on a bone scan a day or two after the initial injury. You can distinguish shinsplints from a stress fracture by a couple of clues. First, in stress fracture, the pain increases abruptly, and second, it's usually concentrated in a smaller area (about one inch in diameter), rather than all along your shinbone, as is the case with shinsplints.

In compartment syndrome, enlarged muscles build up pressure inside muscle compartments (thick, fibrous tubes) of the lower leg. The result can be obstruction of blood supply to lower leg muscles, which can result in serious muscle damage if not treated. Compartment-syndrome pain is felt along the outer front part of the shin. The area is swollen and highly sensitive to touch. See your doctor immediately if the swelling doesn't go down after a few hours.

What to Do for Shinsplints

Wearing athletic shoes with arch supports and adequate cushioning will help to ensure that you're not bothered by shinsplints. Some people may need extra support to prevent excessive pronation (rolling too far onto the inside of your foot as you step on it). Arch supports available off the shelf at a pharmacy or sporting-goods store will probably do the trick. Some people with a more severe problem may need a custom-designed arch support. Warming up before and after exercise is another preventive step for shinsplints—and for other problems as well.

Doctors don't all agree on what to do for the pain of shinsplints. It usually goes away on its own within a couple weeks, but you can do some things that might make you feel more comfortable. Some experimentation may be needed to find what helps you.

For starters, give your lower legs a rest for a while. When the time comes to dive back into your usual activity, start out gently. Cut back your routine, and gradually work up to your normal activity level over the span of a week or so.

Applying an ice massage should help soothe the pain. Rub the area with ice for five to ten minutes, and repeat the process a couple of times a day. (Covering your shin with a damp cloth first will make icing less jarring.) After a few days, when the pain has subsided, you may want to apply moist heat (sit in a hot tub, or apply a warm, wet cloth) for 15 minutes once or twice a day. This can help relax muscles and stimulate blood flow into the region to speed healing.

While you're healing, practice a few simple stretches to improve the flexibility and strength of your lower-leg muscles. Move your foot toward your shin as far as it will go and hold for a few seconds. Repeat several times, as comfortable. Then point the foot away from the front of your leg as far as you can, and again hold for a few seconds and repeat. Next, turn your foot inward and rotate it to the upward position; hold a few seconds and repeat.

Other stretches that will work on your lower-leg muscles include calf stretches. Stand about two feet

Healing the Pain

from a wall, facing it, and step forward about six inches with one leg. Put your hands on the wall in front of you and lean towards it, bending your front leg. You'll feel a stretch in the calf of the back leg. Hold for a few seconds and then do the exercise again, reversing your legs. Another good calf stretch involves getting up on your tiptoes and holding that stance for several seconds. Apply ice to soothe any swelling or pain afterward.

Remember, if you fail to see an improvement in your condition within a few days, it's time to see your doctor to be certain you don't have some other lower-leg problem.

Sore Throat

Ranking right up there with the common cold, a sore throat is one of the most prevalent of human ailments, and the two often travel and arrive together. In fact, a sore throat almost always accompanies some other disease, although it can appear as a solo disorder. To be more precise, there are actually different types of sore throats, with varying causes and symptoms.

Pharyngitis

Pharyngitis is the term doctors use for an infection of the pharynx, the part of the throat that stretches from the tonsils to the voice box. Bacteria or viruses are the usual culprits responsible for the infection. Symptoms include pain when swallowing or speaking, redness, and a feeling of rawness. A fever and swollen lymph glands in your neck may also appear. Pharyngitis often goes along with a cold because the constant postnasal drip irritates the throat, and nasal congestion may force you to

Healing the Pain

breathe through the mouth, causing throat dryness.

Besides being the result of an infection, pharyngitis can also be brought on by overuse of throat muscles or the voice. Sometimes people get a sore throat because of heartburn attacks, when stomach acid backs up into the throat. Allergies can trigger sore throats, which often bring on a scratchy, ticklish sensation. Smoking and drinking alcohol can make a sore throat worse.

Strep throat is the common name for pharyngitis caused by a *Streptococcus* bacteria. Typically it comes on suddenly and brings severe throat pain, perhaps accompanied by headache, fever, nausea, and abdominal pain. Usually there will be no cold symptoms, no cough, and no hoarseness as often exists with pharyngitis caused by viruses or other types of bacteria. Chil-

dren between the ages of 5 and 15 are the most likely to get strep throat. If not treated, strep throat can lead to rheumatic fever.

Tonsillitis

Tonsillitis is an infection of the tonsils, the glands on either side of the throat, which are visible when you open your mouth and look in the mirror. Children are much more likely than adults to get tonsillitis. Symptoms include a sore throat (more painful than the usual pharyngitis), pain upon swallowing, headache, chills, fever, and tonsils that are red and swollen (perhaps also having pus). You might feel swollen glands in the neck and under the jaw.

Laryngitis

Laryngitis is an infection of the larynx, or voice box. If you have laryngitis, you will most likely be hoarse, talking may hurt, and you may lose your voice completely

Healing the Pain

for a while. Laryngitis strikes when your larynx gets irritated because of overuse, smoking, excessive alcohol use, or heartburn (when stomach acids back up into the throat).

What to Do for a Sore Throat

Many cases of sore throat can be safely treated at home. If you have a sore throat that lingers beyond a few days, however, see a doctor to be sure some other health problem isn't involved.

You should also seek medical attention if you suspect your pharyngitis is due to a strep infection. Before prescribing antibiotics for the strep, your doctor should confirm the diagnosis with a culture or antigen test. At this time, penicillin is still the preferred antibiotic for treating strep. It is usually prescribed to be taken orally for 10 days.

All too often, however, people go to the doctor expecting to get a prescription for an antibiotic to cope with any type of sore throat, not just those caused by strep. But the vast majority of sore throat infections are caused by viruses, not bacteria. But antibiotics are only effective against bacteria. Taking an antibiotic for a virus is not only useless in the immediate sense, it can do overall harm in the long run because today's prevalent practice of antibiotic overuse is spurring the development of resistant organisms. If you don't have strep, and your doctor sends you home without an antibiotic, be assured he or she is doing the right thing.

For typical pharyngitis not due to strep, you can help yourself by drinking plenty of liquids in the form of water, fruit juices, broths, or teas. Try to drink at least eight

eight-ounce glasses a day. Taking vitamin C can help. According to some recent medical studies, zinc lozenges may help speed recovery from sore throats and other cold symptoms. You can also try various homemade gargles to soothe your sore throat. A few of these include: salt water (one cup of warm water plus a teaspoon of salt); or warm salt water with a drop of goldenseal tincture added; or a small pinch of cayenne pepper combined with a half-cup of warm water, one tablespoon of lemon juice, and one teaspoon of salt.

Herbal remedies often recommended for sore throat include teas made from ginger or slippery elm. Echinacea and goldenseal are also said to be effective sore-throat remedies. Strong herbal teas made with thyme or sage can be used as a gargle.

If your symptoms indicate you might have tonsillitis, see your doctor. For laryngitis, give your voice a rest and drink lots of liquids. When you must talk, speaking softly is better than whispering; the latter is actually harder on your voice. While some people opt to take aspirin to relieve a sore throat, you should never use aspirin for laryngitis while you are hoarse. The result could be bleeding into the vocal cords, and that could lead to permanent hoarseness.

Tendinitis

Tendinitis is one of the most common afflictions of athletes—amateurs and professionals alike. It may strike you in the elbow after a strenuous game of racquetball, especially if you haven't played for a while. Or you may see an NBA basketball player applying ice to his knees to ward off a case of chronic tendinitis. Sports activities aren't the only irritant, however. People develop tendinitis from activities as diverse as gardening and swinging a roofing hammer eight hours a day.

Tendinitis refers to a tear or an inflammation of a tendon, the band of fibrous tissue that connects muscle to bone. Symptoms include pain (which worsens with activity), swelling, and tenderness in the affected area. The tendons most commonly affected include those in the shoulder, elbow, knee, and heel (where the Achilles tendon is located). Some forms of tendinitis have common household names, such as tennis elbow (when it's on the outside of the elbow) and golfer's elbow (when it strikes the inside of the elbow).

In most cases, the pain will vanish in a few weeks. But someone who's prone to chronic attacks of tendinitis can, over time, do permanent damage to the tendons. If you keep overusing the tendon, tissue will scar, causing diminished flexibility. Tendons and ligaments may stiffen, making movement more difficult. And the older you get, the longer it takes to heal after each bout of tendinitis. In time your tendon may lose its ability to heal, resulting in ongoing pain. If you're repeatedly having problems with tendinitis, your body is telling you to modify your behavior in some way. Perhaps you need to stop a certain activity or do it in a way that puts less stress on your tendon in order to avert irreversible damage.

How do you distinguish tendinitis from the delayed-onset muscle soreness you often get the day after a good workout? You'll feel the latter deep inside the muscle,

Healing the Pain

lasting for only a few days. Tendinitis, on the other hand, is pain at or near the site of the bone-tendon junction, and it will hurt longer. See your doctor if you are unsure as to the source of your muscle soreness.

Recent medical research warns of another cause of tendinitis that has nothing to do with overexertion. Studies have shown that certain antibiotics—a category called fluoroquinolones, used to treat bladder, respiratory, and other infections—can, in rare cases, lead to tendinitis. If the use of medication continues once tendinitis has set in, the tendon may even rupture, requiring surgery. According to researchers, the Achilles tendon at the back of the heel is the most vulnerable. As of summer 1996, consumer advocate groups successfully lobbied the U.S. Food and Drug Administration for warnings on these medications. (European doctors have been warning their patients for years.) But many consumers and doctors may not read the fine print. If you develop tendinitis and take any of these medications, you should alert your doctor: You may be advised to stop use of the drug immediately.

What to Do for Tendinitis

Prompt treatment is crucial to prevent tendinitis from getting worse. One well-accepted therapy is the RICE routine (rest, ice, compression, and elevation). Don't use the painful limb for a few days, and use a sling if you can. Elevating an arm or leg may help control swelling and ease pain. Apply an ice pack to the sore area for no more than 20 minutes on joint areas, where the nerves are close to the surface of the skin. Do this a few times a day. (Covering the area with a moist cloth before applying an ice pack may be more comfortable.) To provide compression, wrap the sore area with an elasticized bandage. Once movement is more comfortable, get back in motion so your joint doesn't stiffen up. After a couple days of ice treatments, switch to heat.

Gentle exercises help to stretch and strengthen muscles. The exact exercises vary according to the location of your tendinitis. Below are just a few examples. A doctor or physical therapist can give you many others.

Tennis elbow. Wrist curls offer a good exercise. Hold a light dumbbell in your hand, with your arm extended by your side, your elbow in a locked position, and your palm facing forward. Gently flex your wrist forward as far as it will go, then release it back to the starting position. Repeat several times. Stop if you feel pain.

Shoulder tendinitis. To strengthen your shoulder, lie on your good side with your painful shoulder up, supporting your head with the other hand. Holding a light weight in your hand—or just the weight of your arm to start with—bend the lower arm of the sore shoulder at a right angle to your body, so it points straight up, but keep the elbow pressed against your side. Slowly lower the weight toward the floor, keeping your elbow touching your side. Raise the weight and repeat no more than ten times, as is comfortable.

Aspirin or other nonsteroidal inflammatory drugs (NSAIDs), including ibuprofen (Advil) and others, can bring relief from pain. For serious cases of tendinitis, your doctor may consider a steroid injection.

Acupuncture may be helpful in cases of chronic tendinitis, and although massage in not advised while pain is present, it may be useful after physical activity to lessen the chance that tendinitis will develop.

To prevent future attacks of tendinitis, keep your muscles in shape and flexible. Always warm up before you exercise. And remember, stretching itself is not a warmup. Stretching cold muscles can lead to injury. Warm up by jogging in place or mimicking the movements of the sport you're about to play (swinging a racquet before a game of tennis, for example). Taking a hot bath is another way to warm up.

Temporo - Mandibular Disorder (TMD)

For temporomandibular joint disorder, or TMD, the diagnostic pendulum has swung from one extreme to the other over the past several decades. At first, TMD (you might recognize it by its former name, temporomandibular joint syndrome, or TMJ) was a condition that no one had ever heard of; then it became the favorite diagnosis of the day for anyone who complained about jaw pain and a host of accompanying symptoms.

Medical experts now are taking a hard look at exactly what TMD is and what to do about it. Still, no definitive answers have been revealed. In fact, considerable disagreement persists about diagnosing and treating TMD.

At the core of the quandary is the temporomandibular joint itself, a tiny disk-shaped joint located in front of each ear that allows us to open and close our mouths. Every day as we talk, eat, yawn, laugh,

and put our jaws through countless other movements, the joints,
bones, muscles, and ligaments
work together in a complex web
of interactions.

But sometimes the jaw joint mal-
functions, causing persistent pain
in the jaw muscles and a host of
other possible problems. If this
happens and you move your lower
jaw, you may hear a grinding,
clicking, or popping sound.
Chewing and talking may be difficult, and you may notice a limita-
tion in the amount you can open
your mouth. Besides pain in the
jaw itself, you may have a
headache, toothache, earache, or a
painful muscle in the face or neck.

No one knows for sure what
causes TMD, although the American Dental Association estimates
that as many as ten million Americans suffer from some form of
temporomandibular disorder. And

TMD strikes women far more
often than men. Some studies
indicate that women account for
as many as 90 percent of TMD
sufferers. Various factors might
contribute to the disorder: teeth-
clenching and grinding, emotional
stress, improper fitting together of
the upper and lower teeth, and a
congenital abnormality. Degenerative diseases, bad posture (such as
habitually carrying a heavy bag on
one shoulder or cradling a phone
between your cheek and shoulder), a blow to the jaw, whiplash,
too much gum-chewing, or eating
too many chewy foods (such as
dried fruits or bagels) also play a
part. But it can be difficult to sort
out which of these are actual
causes and which are merely
aggravating a disorder that already
exists.

The upshot of all this? A person
with chronic jaw pain can be put

through a lot of hoops in searching for a diagnosis. You may need to see a doctor, dentist, and psychologist to get to the bottom of what's causing your pain.

What to Do for TMD

While medical experts still are trying to sort out exactly what TMD is and what causes it, they seem to agree overwhelmingly on one point: Treatment of the disorder should be conservative. That was the message of a consensus conference on TMD convened in May 1996 by the National Institutes of Health (NIH). Clearly, too many people have spent far too much money on TMD treatments that not only didn't work, but also resulted in more pain—or worse.

For instance, back in the 1970s and 1980s, thousands of TMD sufferers underwent surgery to receive jaw implants. A specially-coated disk was inserted in the jaw joint to act as a sort of shock absorber. But the natural pressures of chewing caused these implants to disintegrate, setting off biochemical reactions that wore away the jawbone. The implant device eventually was taken off the market, but by then many people faced repeated surgeries to repair the damage. Many of those who had been treated were left permanently disabled or disfigured.

If any health care provider recommends that you have surgery for TMD, get a second opinion, and perhaps a third. Some experts today believe surgery is never appropriate for TMD. And almost all agree that if surgery is used at all, it should only be undertaken as a last resort.

When the NIH consensus conference panel called for a "conservative" approach to TMD therapy, they were advocating treatments that create no permanent change in the jaw structure or position and thus do not require jaw surgery.

Fortunately, a number of self-care practices are available that can help eliminate or at least reduce the pain from TMD:

- Dietary changes. Try a softer diet, and stop chewing gum.
- Cold or heat. A cold compress on the affected area may ease the pain. Some people, however, think moist heat works better. Experiment to see which works better for you. You may want to try alternating cold and heat.
- Stress management. If you think stress plays a role in your TMD, learn techniques for keeping stress under control. Try to avoid grinding your teeth or clenching your jaw in response to stress.
- Exercise. Gentle exercises that relax jaw and neck muscles can

be enormously helpful. A simple one is the head roll, which calls for gentle rolling of the head in a circular motion—first to the right, then to the left. A physical therapist would be able to advise you on additional relaxation exercises.

- Habit evaluation. Analyze habitual movements that may be contributing to your TMD, such as clenching your teeth or chewing on pencils.
- Over-the-counter medications. If you need additional pain relief, you could try taking acetaminophen (Tylenol). Other pain relievers that can also be helpful include aspirin or other NSAIDs (nonsteroidal anti-inflammatory drugs), such as ibuprofen (Advil).
- Acupressure. Pressure on various acupoints may help relieve TMD pain. For example, one such point is known as ST6, located

between the lower jaw and skull. To locate it, clench your teeth and feel for the tightened jaw muscle between your lower jaw and skull. Firmly press on the ST6 points with your fingers on both sides of the head. Breathe slowly and deeply. Hold the pressure for about two minutes. You might also benefit from acupuncture. Contact a qualified acupuncturist to discuss treatment.

Healing the Pain

INDEX

Anxiety
  acupuncture and, 9
  back pain and, 158
  biofeedback and, 23
  cancer pain and, 164
  chest pain and, 173
  fibromyalgia and, 189
  hypnosis and, 68
  massage and, 77
  support groups and, 130, 134
Applied kinesiology, 32
Arthritis. *See also* Gout;
      Osteoarthritis; Rheumatoid
      arthritis.
  acupuncture and, 9
  biofeedback and, 24
  bursitis and, 162
  chiropractic and, 33
  cold/heat treatments and, 42,
      45, 157
  exercise and, 50–52, 156
  fibromyalgia, compared to,
      189–190
  herbal medicine and, 62
  NSAIDs and, 96, 121, 156
  TENS and, 147
  treatment, 156–157
  types, 154–155
  variabilities of, 155–156
Aspiration percutaneous lumbar
      diskectomy, 142
Aspirin (acetylsalicylic acid)
  arthritis and, 156
  benefits of, 96
  cancer pain and, 167
  chest pain and, 174
  contraindications, 97, 231
  headaches and, 197
  menstrual cramps and, 205
  risks of, 97–98
  tendinitis and, 235

Aspirin (continued)
  TMD and, 239
Asthma, 9, 23, 33, 98
Atherosclerosis, 173
Ayurvedic medicine, 57

Ɓ
Back pain. *See also* Low back pain.
  biofeedback and, 23
  causes of, 35, 158–159
  cold/heat treatments and, 45,
      161
  exercise for, 48–50, 159, 160
  herbal medicine and, 62
  incidence of, 157
  massage and, 76
  OTC medications and, 91
  physical therapy and, 115, 116,
      160
  prevention, 159–160
  surgery for, 140–142
  treatment, 160–161
Baclofen (Lioresal), 212
Bedside pain medication pumps,
      125–126
Beta blockers, 174
Biofeedback
  chest pain and, 174
  choosing practitioners, 27
  credibility of, 26
  fibromyalgia and, 24, 191
  headaches and, 24, 197
  history of, 22
  physical therapy and, 113
  physiological effects of, 21–23
  research studies, 24–26
  side effects, 26–27
  uses/applications, 23–26
Bladder infections, 33
Bonica, John, 108
Braces and splints, 160, 171

Healing the Pain

N

Nafarelin acetate, 184
Naproxen sodium (Aleve), 91, 96,
    149–150, 151, 156, 163, 193
Narcotics, 121–122
Nausea and vomiting
    acupuncture and, 9
    from chemotherapy, 70
    chest pain and, 173
    migraines and, 121
    narcotics and, 121
    ovarian cysts and, 213
Neck pain
    biofeedback and, 23
    causes of, 35
    exercise for, 53–55
    massage and, 76
    nerve blocks and, 88
    TMD and, 144, 236
Nerve blocks
    adverse effects, 88–89
    cancer pain and, 86, 167
    categories, 82–83
    contraindications, 87
    functions of, 84–85
    postherpetic neuralgia and, 88,
        213
    techniques, 83
    uses/applications, 86–89
Nerve (injury) pain. See also Carpal
        tunnel syndrome; Herniated
        (slipped) disks; Neuralgia.
    acupuncture and, 9
    antidepressants and, 122–123
    chymopapain and, 143
    herbal medicine and, 64
    nerve blocks and, 86
    prescription medication for, 124
    TENS and, 151, 212
    treatment, 211–213
    types/causes, 209–211

Nettles, 62, 64
Neuralgia. See also Facial neuralgia;
        Trigeminal neuralgia.
    defined, 209
    herbal medicine and, 64
    nerve blocks and, 89
    prescription medications and,
        122
    TENS and, 147, 212
Neurolytic blocks, 82–83, 86
Nitroglycerin, 174
Nonneurolytic blocks, 83
Nonprescription medications. See
        Over-the-counter (OTC)
        medications.
Nonsteroidal anti-inflammatory
        drugs (NSAIDs). See also
        Aspirin (acetylsalicylic acid);
        Ibuprofen; Indomethacin;
        Naproxen sodium.
    actions of, 95–96, 121
    benefits of, 96
    brand name vs. generic, 91
    risks of, 97–98, 121
    uses/applications, 91, 197
Norepinephrine, 77
Novocain, 176
NSAIDs. See Nonsteroidal anti-
        inflammatory drugs.
Numbness, sensation of, 53, 158,
        168, 196, 209
Nuprin. See Ibuprofen.

O

Occupational therapy
    choosing practitioners, 118
    defined, 111
    described, 116
    methods in, 116–118
    physical therapy, compared to,
        111–112

Healing the Pain

Healing the Pain

Healing the Pain

Tension headaches (*continued*)
  nerve blocks and, 88
  symptoms, 195
  treatment, 197–198
Thyme, 231
Thyroid hormone, 169
Tic douloureux. *See* Trigeminal
    neuralgia.
Tingling, sensation of, 53, 168, 196
Tinnitus
  aspirin, NSAIDs and, 98
  biofeedback and, 24
  ear pain and, 179, 181
  TENS and, 148
TMD. *See* Temporomandibular joint
    disorder.
Tonsillitis, 229–230, 231
Toothaches. *See* Dental pain.
Traction, physical therapy and, 114
Transcutaneous electrical nerve
    stimulation (TENS)
  cancer pain and, 147, 167
  cautions, 148–149
  defined, 146–147
  dental pain and, 147, 177
  individual responses to, 152
  low back pain and, 151
  menstrual cramps and, 151
  nerve pain and, 212
  osteoarthritis and, 149–150
  in pain clinics, 106
  peripheral nerve pain and, 212
  physical therapy and, 114
  postsurgical pain and, 148, 221
  research studies, 149–152
  shingles and, 224–225
  techniques, 146–147
  uses/applications, 147–148
Transdermal patches, 124
Trigeminal neuralgia, 9, 210–211,
    212–213

Trigger points, 81, 86–87
Tylenol. *See* Acetaminophen
    (Tylenol).

U
Ulcers, 35, 97
Ultrasound, 44

V
Vaginal pain, 70
Valerian, 63, 64, 204
Varicella-zoster virus, 221
Vision problems, 10, 33, 196
Vitamin B_6, 171
Vitamin C, 231
Vitamin deficiency, peripheral
    neuropathy and, 209
Vitex, 63
Vomiting. *See* Nausea and vomiting.

W
Weed, Samuel, 31
Weight, body
  arthritis and, 156
  back pain and, 158, 159, 160
  carpal tunnel syndrome and,
    169, 171
  chest pain and, 174
  gout and, 191–192, 194
  heartburn and, 174
Whiplash, 68, 76, 88
White willow bark, 62, 65
Wormwood, 174
Wounds and bruises, 65

Y
Yellow dock root, 63
Yin and yang, 8
Yoga, 54, 205

Z
Zinc lozenges, 231

Healing the Pain

Photo credits:

Front cover: **SuperStock**

FPG International: Paul Ambrose: 11; Ron Chapple: 25, 134;
Jim Cummins: 55, 73, 84; Mark Harmel: 23; Spencer Jones: 57;
Dick Luria: 131; David McGlynn: 71; Jeffery Myers: 36;
Terry Qing: 124; Ken Reid: 60, 119; Robert Reiff: 77;
Stephen Simpson: 30; **Frank Garner/The Stock Market:** 39;
International Stock: Hal Kern: 90; Ronn Maratea: 114, 116;
John Michael: 105; Bill Stanton: 21; Jay Thomas: 43;
Caroline Wood: 79; **Photri:** 86; **Patrick Ryan/TENS Elpha 2000
Courtesy of Care Rehab, McLean, Virginia:** 146;
SuperStock: 47, 51, 52, 80, 96, 101, 106, 113, 127, 137, 138.

Healing the Pain

Robin